Surviving Pancreatic Cancer

Your Guide to Life

Larisa Belote

Surviving Pancreatic Cancer

Step by Step - Wellness
4 Bridge Plaza Drive
Manalapan, NJ 07726
http://www.stepbystep-wellness.com/

The content of this book is for general instruction only. Each person's physical, emotional, and spiritual condition is unique. The instruction in this book is not intended to replace or interrupt the reader's relationship with a physician or other professional. Please consult your doctor for matters pertaining to your specific health and diet.

Edited and formatted by Andy Letke

Belote, Larisa.
    Surviving Pancreatic Cancer : Your Guide to Life / Larisa Belote. ~~ 1st ed.

    ISBN: 978-0-9962662-0-8

Printed in the United States of America

First Edition

In loving memory of my mom…

Thank you for being there every step of the way
We knew we could count on you always
You were a loving mother, this we all know and felt
Till the last minute, you gave a piece of yourself
People you touched, the smile you left behind
You will always be in our hearts and in our minds

Surviving Pancreatic Cancer Your Guide to Life

by Larisa Belote

Contents

Acknowledgements

I am very lucky to have many wonderful and caring people in my life that give me support, guidance and a whole lot of love. I would like to thank everyone who contributed his or her time and effort in making this book possible.

To my dear husband: Thank you for being very patient and supportive through the book writing process. Your love helped me get through many sad and emotional days.

To Andy Letke, my wonderful editor: Thank you for spending endless hours on editing my writing and helping me with all aspects of the book. Your dedication is truly incredible!

To my loving children: Thanks for being there when I needed you most.

To my father and brothers: You are all very dear to me and very close to my heart. I love you!

Introduction

Hi! My name is Larisa and I want you to meet my mom, Raya, right there in the picture on the right. This book is about Raya, who is a pancreatic cancer survivor. This is not a biography. This is a story about a 54-year-old woman who was diagnosed with Stage IV metastatic pancreatic cancer, was given 3 months to live, but instead survived. Was in total remission in 6 months and lived a good quality of life for 17 years after.

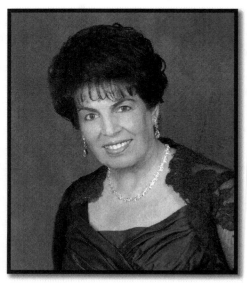

Pancreatic cancer was and still is a deadly disease. To this day, there is still no real cure for this terminal illness that has taken numerous lives very quickly without sparing any pain. Stage IV metastatic cancer is the last on the list of staged cancers. It has not only attacked and taken over the pancreas, but spread to the adjoining organs. From this point there was no return or so mom was told.

Based on statistics, doctors gave mom three months to live with chemotherapy or radiation treatment option that would prolong mom's life by only one month with a very painful and dreadful side effects. Mom decided to decline the traditional treatments that were offered and put trust in her children to do research and find holistic and innovative treatments that had saved her life.

It took a lot of courage and discipline, but with the help and support of her family, Mom made a drastic life style change. She nourished her body with food and juices that helped rebuild her strength and boost the immune system. She took various supplements and had IV vitamin infusions on a regular basis. And most importantly, underwent body radiosurgery which was an innovative precise radiation treatment.

At 54, mom was still young and had a whole life ahead of her. She had a loving husband, 3 beautiful grown children and 2 very adorable grandchildren. She was young and still had many dreams and desires to fulfill. But cancer did not care. Cancer does not wait for you to be ready and to be old. It can strike at any age, any time and place. It is not only common here in the US, but all over the world.

My mom was the type of person that was selfless. She would take care of everyone else first and then herself. Even when she was young, she always put her parents' needs before her own. For most of her life, she lived in the city of Samarkand, former Soviet Union, with her two brothers and four sisters. She was the youngest of the family, but the smartest and the prettiest in my opinion. She had a very hard life growing up in a big family with a small income. Even though she helped her father with his business at a very young age, she made sure to educate herself in a university and became a trauma nurse.

Later on she got married and had children. She was a dedicated wife and mother. She worked and took care of her three children while her husband worked as a pilot with odd hours and hardly had time to help her. She raised her children well and always made sure they had a homemade meal and were always dressed in clean clothes. After all, at that time there were no washing machines that performed all the functions as they do now. Washing machine would wash the clothing, but since there was no spin cycle, clothes had to be wrung out by hand and hung to dry either outside if the weather was permitting on clothing lines and held by clothespins or hung inside the apartment.

In the summer of 1979, my family along with my mom's brother's families and my grandmother immigrated to the United States. It was a hard transition, but none the less it happened. We moved to Brooklyn and lived there for ten years with my maternal grandmother. As much as mom wanted to go to school in order to get her nursing license, it was not possible. Her responsibility laid with the care she needed to give to her mother and her children.

After my grandmother passed away in 1985, mom trained to be nurse's aide. She worked in nursing homes for a while and later, to ease the hard physical labor, found a job in a warehouse where she worked as an office manager.

In 1996, mom was diagnosed with very harsh and incurable disease, pancreatic cancer. It was very devastating to all of us. It was very hard to imagine life without our dearest mother. We were a very close knit family, and mom kept everyone together like glue. She was full of life and laughter and kept all her family smiling at all times.

This book is a story about my mom, but it is also A Guide to Life. You will find this guide at the end of the book. It is there to help you better understand the necessary dietary changes that would be helpful to make in order to heal the body. It lists the holistic approaches to therapies and treatment options that helped my mom in the recovery process. I hope this information will be helpful and useful.

My goal is to bring awareness to pancreatic cancer. It's about giving people the confidence and motivation to get better even if they are at the very advanced stages of cancer. Don't give up hope! Instead, educate and empower your soul with knowledge about the disease and find treatments that will prolong life, not only to exist but to live a good quality of life with your loved ones.

As you enter the journey of Surviving Pancreatic Cancer, I hope you will be inspired to make a change in your life. Then, touch a life of someone else in need and as the time goes on, create a ripple effect in the world.

Chapter 1:

The Phone Call to Reality

The phone rang. This was the call that I had been waiting for—the call that would tell me if my mother would live or die. This was the call that would confirm whether the biopsy was benign or malignant. At that point, I was not sure if I wanted to know, but I had no choice. I needed to know. I answered and listened. After I heard that my mom's biopsy was positive and it was confirmed that it was, indeed, cancer, my mind went into a complete fog as tears rolled down my cheeks. I could not speak; it felt like there was a big stone in my throat. After hanging up, I wondered how this could be possible. This was not fair as my mom was so young. At 54, she had not lived her life fully and had not seen her grandchildren grow up. There were still so many things to do.

As my feet began to tremble, I laid down in my bed and cried uncontrollably. Many thoughts entered my mind. What's next? Is there a cure for this wretched disease? How long does my mom have to live? How am I going to tell my father and my brothers that my mom has pancreatic cancer? How am I going to face my mother and reveal to her that she has a terminal illness? Lying there, I stared at the wall for what seemed like an eternity, but I eventually fell asleep.

Opening my eyes and surging up to a sitting position, I looked at the clock noticing it was already morning. I rolled my feet off the bed and onto the floor heading for the window. The sun had risen and it was just another day. How could that be? I felt so betrayed. When I heard that my mom had pancreatic cancer, everything stopped moving. I thought there was not going to be another day, not going to be another sunrise, the clock would stop ticking, and time would stand still. As far as I was concerned, the world stopped living. After all, the dearest person in my life now had a life sentence. Though looking through the window, it seemed that all my thoughts were wrong. The sun did rise and it was just another ordinary day. Life did not stop and kept on moving. I had to face reality and continue living.

Chapter 2:

Finding out the Diagnosis

My mom had not been feeling well for a while now. She complained of pain on her left side most of the time after she ate. She said that whenever she ate anything, it seemed like it was going to that particular spot—it felt like a rock that wouldn't move. To alleviate the constant pain, she took Tylenol. After a long while, the pain would subside. Food was her worst enemy: pain, pain, pain after she ate! It was just better to stay hungry, but she needed food to survive and have energy. So, she would eat again and go through the same vicious cycle. By this time, Mom lost twenty-one pounds. She was frail and weak. She couldn't do much without taking frequent breaks to catch her breath and rest. Her internal medicine practitioner was concerned about the weight loss, but thought it was good since she was always a little overweight.

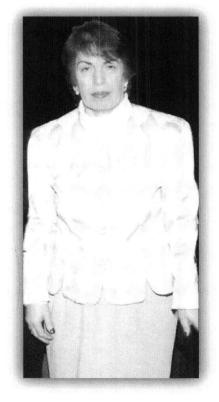

Mom's doctor was very thorough and always went through her medical history with new questions. He sent my mom to some of the wonderful specialists within his circle. For starters, she went for relevant blood tests. He also felt that she needed to see a gastroenterologist who performed an endoscopy and a colonoscopy, both of which came back normal. After she was losing too much weight, he sent her for a CAT scan, blood work, and other tests, but nothing was out of the ordinary and always came back normal. Everyone in my family thought the lack of results was very strange. She didn't have any major medical problems in the past except for heavy bleeding during her periods, which was due to fibroids in the uterus. The only surgery she had was a total hysterectomy about three years prior due to massive blood loss and debilitating cramps during menstruation, which caused severe anemia. The surgeon thought it was best to remove both the uterus and the ovaries at the time, which I didn't have any opinion over and thought it would be best in order to help my mom overcome the problem.

Now, since I have gained knowledge, I realize that the hysterectomy probably wasn't the best decision considering it put my mom into menopause, which caused many issues physically and in her intimate life. I continue to think that if I had researched other possible treatments for excessive bleeding and fibroids that I might have saved my mom from going through a hysterectomy.

At that time, I was recuperating from a C-section from the birth of my oldest son. I was very busy learning to be a mom, looking after a baby, and managing my household. I also nursed the baby, which seemed to be an endless task. By the time I was done with one feeding, it would be time for the next one. Believe me, even though it sounds like I am complaining, I really enjoyed those moments. The only issue was that I didn't have the chance to concentrate on my mom because of my newly added responsibilities. I didn't have all of the solutions anyway. I thought that the doctors knew best, so I agreed to their suggestions. I am not saying that all doctors are the same, but I learned that you have to stop for a moment and think whether the suggested treatment is the correct one for you. Would the situation have been different had my mom not done the hysterectomy? Now, it probably does not matter. What's done is done. It's in the past. We live and learn, and hopefully the next decision made will be with much learned knowledge.

Anyway, a couple of months after the hysterectomy, the gynecologist put my mom on a synthetic hormone, ***Premarin***, to help with menopausal symptoms. Some of her symptoms got better. I would have approached that decision differently now, but I'll save that story for another book. I'd like to give you a brief synopsis about Premarin so that you know exactly what the source is and how it affects women in the long run.

Premarin is a patented horse hormone made from equilin, which is pregnant mare's urine and it contains only estrogen. A reproductive woman naturally makes estrogen every day of the month and progesterone two weeks of each month. If a woman takes Premarin, not only is she taking a substance that is foreign to her body, but she also is not taking progesterone to balance the estrogen. This can be dangerous to the human body…it's a possible cancer setup. The molecular structure of Premarin is different from that of a human-produced hormone, which is not compatible with the horse's estrogen. The side effects of Premarin are potentially devastating. Pemarin raises the C-reactive protein, the one absolute marker for heart attack. Cardiologists routinely check women who take Premarin monitoring this marker. If the marker is high, the doctor would prescribe the drug Lipitor.[1]

One evening my mom was in a lot of pain. She drank Tylenol, which didn't take the pain away. I called just in time, so I asked my father to take her to the ER to get some relief. I was not sure what they could do for her, but it was worth a try. Maybe they would find out why her pain level was so high. While they were on their way to the ER, I raced from NJ to meet them at the hospital. I lived with my husband and two little kids about an hour and a half from my parents, which made times like these very hard to manage.

I arrived at the ER and found my parents still in the waiting room two hours later. The nurse saw her already, but they were waiting for one of the rooms to be available. Meanwhile she was still in pain and had taken more Tylenol. About an hour later, they escorted her to a stretcher in the hallway because all the other areas had other patients. The doctor eventually paid us a visit. After I explained that my mom had a lot of pain on one side of her abdomen and that the Tylenol didn't help her much, he gave her a much stronger pain reliever to subside the pain. He also assigned a blood test and an abdominal CAT scan, which required her to drink a certain fluid so they could see the organs better during the test.

We were exhausted waiting at the hospital wondering if the sun had yet risen. I thought I would collapse considering my feet were in so much pain from standing the entire time. About four hours after they put my mom on a stretcher in the hallway, they finally wheeled her into an area with other patients separated by curtains. I made a beeline for the chair next to the bed and sank into it. My father paced in and out of the waiting room. At least one of us was able to rest the feet.

The professionals finished all of the tests and we waited patiently for the results. About an hour later, the doctor came to talk to us. He said the blood work and the CAT scan were both normal and he wanted us to go home and contact the internist if the pain persisted. I asked the doctor, "If all the tests are showing nothing, then why is my mom in so much pain? Why has she lost so much weight and can hardly eat anything without experiencing pain thirty minutes after meals?" I was tired of getting the same answer all the time, "It's nothing—everything looks fine."

According to the test results, the doctor said that she was fine and there was nothing he could do right then except prescribe pain medication. I was furious, as was my mom. My mom said, "So I should be taking pain medication for the rest of my life? That's it?" The doctor looked very tired and just wanted to leave the room. I didn't want him to leave until we got some closure and found out what was causing all of the pain. Unfortunately, the doctor had to leave without giving any diagnosis except for saying that maybe it was just indigestion. I wanted to scream. How many times did we have to hear that no one has an answer? Meanwhile, my mom's condition was getting worse. We took Mom home with the same heavy feeling as before, knowing that we still had no answer.

The next day, I contacted a family friend who also happens to be an internal medicine doctor that my mom used when she lived in Brooklyn. I wanted to fill him in on what was going on with my mom. His practice was in Brooklyn and I didn't want to bother him before, but I had no one else to turn to for answers. He was a very good physician with very bright colleagues and a referral pool of specialists and other physicians. I briefly explained to him my mom's pain, the weight loss, and the tests that were completed. Although he was talking to me calmly, I could hear the heavy breathing on the other end. He asked me to bring the emergency room CAT scan to the radiologist he worked with and the blood tests to his office. I was able to go to the hospital with my mom's hand-written release form to pick up the CAT scan films and bring them to the radiologist by that afternoon.

An hour-and-a-half later, I got a phone call from the internist. He said that the radiologist reviewed the films and he noticed that there was a very large growth in the tail of the pancreas, which was very apparent. The internist and his radiologist were both appalled that the ER radiologist missed the growth on the CAT scan from just the night before. I was shocked, furious, and sad because my mom was probably not the only one that radiologist misdiagnosed. I know ER doctors work long shifts, which can lead to exhaustion, but patients should not have to put their lives in the hands of unfocused and tired physicians in emergency situations or at any time for that matter.

I was just glad that, finally, for better or worse, there was an answer for my mom's pain. The internist urged me to schedule a biopsy of the growth as soon as possible. He didn't want to think the worst, that it might be malignant, and said that it might just be pancreatitis. I know he tried to calm me, but my body got as cold as ice and I was shaking as soon as I heard about the growth in the pancreas. I didn't know what to make of this new information as I was in shock. I resolved to remain optimistic.

Once I processed all the information from that phone call and I stopped being angry, I thought of my mom. The next logical step would be to call and tell her that the ER doctor made a mistake reading the CAT scan. I would have to tell her that the results were not normal and things were not ok—that the doctor overlooked a large growth. My mom had a medical background working as a trauma nurse for many years. Because of this, I knew that questions would pour in regarding the details of the growth that I would not be able to answer. Finally, we had an answer. So many agonizing months slipped by without knowing why she was experiencing so much pain, challenge with eating, and weight loss. The answer was not complete, but it was a start.

I picked up the phone and was about to call her, but realized this information was really going to make her upset. I then hung up the phone and decided to just drive to Queens to tell her in person.

It was a long drive to Queens. It took me almost two hours, but I made my time productive. I phoned people who needed to know laying some groundwork. The first call was to my parents to let them know I was on my way to visit them. I also called my brothers to make sure they could come by for support once I got there. My sister-in-law was next on the list—I asked her about a reliable hospital to do the biopsy.

Although my mom was always happy to see me, she was surprised that I didn't give her much notice for the visit, which didn't leave her sufficient time to prepare. By that, I mean prepare a meal so that we could all sit down at a table and catch up on our happenings, make sure the house was in tip-top shape, and to make sure she looked her best. Even though this visit was not going to be pleasant, I always looked forward to seeing my parents and spending time with them.

I walked inside the house after my father gave me a kiss and a big hug and looked for my mom. She was in the kitchen hovering over the stove cooking. The kitchen was her favorite place in the house because she loved to cook. I looked at her holding back the tears and gave her a kiss and a big hug. I took over the cooking and we spoke casually about the kids, my brothers, and so on for about half an hour waiting for my brothers to arrive.

Mom looked pale and thinner than the last time I saw her. She was moving and doing everything in slow motion conserving her strength. Even though she was smiling, I know she was just doing that to make me happy so that I would not worry about her. I saw that she was not well and probably in pain; she never let the pain bother her or stand in the way of her family unless it was unbearable. She must have taken pain medication to make this visit possible. She seemed to be in good spirits and, as usual, happy to see everyone together at the house. We sat down about an hour after I arrived and ate dinner as a family while having the usual interesting discussions—that passed time until dessert.

Dessert was the most opportune time for me to tell everyone the information I discovered that day. Moving into the living room, we found comfort from the sofa, chairs, and sweet food while I was dreading what I was about to say. My mom sat next to me. I took her hand and turned to her. I looked at everyone else and said that I heard some news today from a different doctor about the CAT scan findings. I know I had everyone's attention; it was quiet and everyone looked at me with frozen faces. I told them that I had spoken to the internal medicine doctor and he confirmed that his radiologist saw a growth in the pancreas, but they were not sure what the diagnosis would be until the biopsy was done. Apparently, the radiologist in the ER made a huge mistake when he said everything looked normal. My mom squeezed my hand very tightly and then burst into tears with whatever strength she had left. I gave her a hug and tried to calm her down by saying that the doctor thinks it might be pancreatitis. I told her not to worry and to be optimistic. At least we knew why she was in pain and losing weight. While I was hugging my mom, I could see everyone else's angry face around the room. "He made a mistake? How could that be?" one said. The other said, "Who was that radiologist? I am going to go there tomorrow and kill him! How could he make such a mistake?" My father just stared at me with a blank face. He was in shock. I remember having the same reaction when I first heard about the new information. I am still upset at the incompetency of the radiologist in the ER.

I tried to calm my family down and let them know that being angry is okay, but it's not going to get us anywhere. Now that we know, we can move on and find out exactly what is wrong with Mom and, perhaps, find a treatment that will help her feel better. They looked at me like I was crazy, but after a while of going back and forth, screaming in disbelief, and trying to make sense of how and why the mistake could have been made, everyone calmed down and we started deriving a plan.

I told everyone about my conversation with my sister-in-law regarding the best possible facility to do a biopsy. I explained that since she worked at Robert Wood Johnson University Hospital

(RWJ), from her experience, she could vouch that it was a good hospital and that the doctors were competent. Of course, we discussed considering a facility closer to home like Long Island University Hospital, North Shore University Hospital, or even some hospitals in New York City. Not only did we need to figure out which hospital would facilitate the biopsy, but we also needed to think ahead. Many questions surfaced, like, "What if the outcome was worse than expected?" We had to make sure that there was a good oncology center with good oncologists.

My sister-in-law suggested the Cancer Institute of NJ (CINJ), which is part of RWJ, if it had to be in New Jersey. It would be best to have access to all the records and doctors in one place. We also needed to decide who would have time to take Mom during the week for appointments and give her the care that she needs—to keep in touch with the doctors and to make decisions. My father worked. Ideally, he could take time off, but with the language barrier, this was not a good idea. Both of my brothers worked, but could take a day here or there if necessary. I worked as well and could take a couple of days off if I needed to, but I couldn't travel from New Jersey to Queens often with two little kids at home even though I had a babysitter. I had to be closer to home if I was to be mom's primary caretaker.

After a long discussion, I turned to my mom and asked her which hospital she would rather go to and where would she feel more comfortable. She looked at me with tears in her eyes and said that she completely trusts us as a family to make this decision and she will follow. She didn't want to bring any hardship to any of us. She just wanted us to live our lives happily. This time, the happy part was not possible, at least not for now. We just wanted to do what was right: choose the best hospital so she could be taken care of properly and given a correct diagnosis so we could move forward and figure out the next step.

All of us felt the pain that she was feeling. We knew that she was a happy person, who took care of all of us and always looked for ways to make everyone else happy around her. Now it was our turn to take care of her, make the right decisions, and in turn, make her happy. By the end of the day, we decided that RWJ was the right choice. I was going to make an appointment with an oncologist recommended by my sister-in-law at CINJ and schedule a biopsy. I went home that night having a good feeling about the decision that we made as a family hoping it would bring us peace soon enough.

With the help of my sister-in-law, I was able to schedule an appointment with the oncologist in less than a week. Usually for new patients there is a much longer wait for an appointment. It definitely pays to know someone, I thought. When my mom and I came to see Dr. Elizabeth Poplin, Medical Oncologist, we were very impressed.

A nurse took my mom's blood pressure, temperature, and weight before the doctor came in the room. Once Dr. Poplin came in, she took her time and went over mom's medical history very thoroughly. She asked when Mom started to lose weight, when the pain began, and how severe it was. She asked about mom's diet and if she was able to eat. Dr. Poplin's voice was very soft, soothing, and as I could see, agreed with my mom.

She performed a comprehensive physical exam on my mom. She examined mom's abdomen, her neck for enlarged lymph nodes, her eyes, and at her skin for any yellow color looking for jaundice. Dr. Poplin stepped out of the room to place orders for three tests, then walked in a couple of minutes later. She ordered special blood work and a complete chest and abdomen CAT scan to assess the condition of the lungs, liver, and other vital organs. She also ordered a biopsy of the affected area in the pancreas. The doctor further explained that a biopsy was necessary to determine if the mass (I called it a growth before) was benign or not. If the mass was not benign, then they needed to stage the disease. We would then need to come back to see Dr. Poplin when the results of the biopsy and blood work were ready.

Upon arriving for the biopsy, I could see that my mom was nervous. She was trying to hide it not to worry me. I think I was more nervous than she was. I was hoping it would be an easy process so she could simply go home in peace without pain, but I was just kidding myself. I knew that it was not going to be pain free—not going to be easy. She was already in pain and now this was going to cause her more pain. The only comforting thought was that after the biopsy we would know the diagnosis, which hopefully would shed some light on the pain my mom had for the longest time.

She walked slowly with me hand in hand into the hospital. A nurse briefed us about the biopsy procedure, changed her into the proper hospital garments, and inserted an intravenous line for fluids. When the nurse was finished, I looked at my mom and gave her a big hug holding my tears back. She looked at me and said, "I am not worried. I just want to know what is wrong with me." Then she walked inside with the nurses.

As I sat waiting for the test to finish, I heard noises from my mom's room. They were loud thumping and banging sounds. I wondered what those noises could have been. In my head, I ran through the procedural steps the nurse discussed with my mom and me. The nurse would administer a local anesthetic to numb the area so my mom would not feel any pain where the radiologist would be working. She was supposed to feel only pressure during the procedure. It was supposed to be a needle biopsy, where, under imaging guidance, a doctor would insert a needle into the mass to remove some tissue. Then a pathologist would examine the tissue under a microscope right there in the room. The rest of the tissue would be sent out to a lab for further testing. This procedure did not sound complicated—painful, but not complicated.

The noises made me nervous. They sounded so loud. For a moment, a door opened to the room, so I jumped up to look in. The doors were heavy and closed very slowly. It looked like my mom was lying down on a table and the person administering the biopsy was inserting the needle quickly up and down, which looked quite painful. The door shut and I could not figure out or see where the noise was coming from. My heart was pounding as I saw the whole thing. My mom was fully awake for this procedure. I guess I would find out all the details when the process was over, which I hoped was soon. The procedure took about an hour.

Finally, a nurse wheeled my mom out of the room and brought her into a different room. There she spent another two hours under the observation of nurses who wanted to make sure she was okay before sending her home. After some time, I was able to speak with her. She was weak, but confirmed that she was in some pain as the anesthetic wore off. She said that she didn't really see what was happening to her during the procedure, but felt heavy pressure. She was happy it was over and ready to go home. A nurse gave us instructions on how to treat the punctured area, warned that there might be some risk of infection, and then discharged my mom. The pathology tests would be ready in about a week.

I drove Mom back to my house. For a couple of days following the procedure, Mom complained of pain in the affected area, but I made sure to change the dressing with bacitracin and it healed well.

A week later, I took my mom to see Dr. Poplin at the CINJ to go over the blood tests and biopsy results. Upon arrival, a receptionist escorted us to a conference room and asked us to sit down in two of the many chairs that surrounded the long rectangular table. On the other side of the long table, other people were sitting and talking to what looked like doctors in white coats. I could not hear their conversation as they spoke inaudibly to keep it private.

A gentleman walked into the room wearing a white coat. Tall, handsome with brownish skin, and a very happy smile on his face, he looked at us asking if this was actually my mom. Discovering that she was the patient he needed to find, the doctor introduced himself. He had great excitement in his voice as if he had good news for us. His attitude allowed me to breathe with ease and have some positive thoughts. My mom sat there looking at him with a smile, encouraged that good news was coming. He did not sit down and spoke very loudly with excitement and happiness exuding from his face. He said, "Raya, we got your pathology report back with the biopsy results. You have stage IV pancreatic cancer, and you have three months to live."

I froze in my chair. A loud ringing occurred in my ears and I could not hear any other words the doctor uttered. The diagnosis just rang repeatedly in my head—pancreatic cancer…stage IV…three months to live…pancreatic cancer…stage IV…three months to live. I looked at my mom and saw that her face was bright red as if she was on fire. I wanted to take her hand into mine, but found that I couldn't move. The doctor continued talking, but I still couldn't hear him. I was in shock. I looked at Mom again and saw tears rolling down her cheeks. She was staring at the doctor's face without any body movement or any change in her facial expression. She was in shock as well.

All of a sudden, I snapped out of whatever shock I was in and felt the adrenaline going through my veins. I was boiling and overwhelmed with anger. How could a person who calls himself a doctor walk in with a smile and have such excitement in his voice telling my mom she has three months to live? I understand that he probably does this all the time and his job is to tell patients their diagnoses, but don't you think he should have had the decency to sit down and prepare my mom (or any other patient, for that matter) for what is to come? I realized that, to him, my mom was probably just a number in his file—just another patient with a terminal illness that he had to divulge the diagnosis. I wanted to shake him. I wanted to tell him just to stop talking and think about how he should be presenting this diagnosis. Maybe he should have consulted me first on my mom's condition and how she was going to take this diagnosis, and then both of us could have eased her into it. We could have told her that her test results don't look so good, that she is sick, and that the illness is a serious one, which has progressed and may not be curable. We could have told her that she may not have a long time to live. We could have told her any other way than the way he just blurted it out—straight and to the point. You are dying. I think the way he presented it just killed her.

Chapter 3:

Treatment Options Given by Doctors and Survival Rates

We were in the conference room for another thirty minutes until both my mom and I could get up off our chairs. As instructed, we walked into Dr. Poplin's office where she went over the pathology report and the blood test findings. She was very calm and chose her words carefully. You could definitely see the years of experience and the gentle way she spoke with patients. By this time, my mom and I were primed. We were ready to hear anything that came at us after that total kill. She explained that the doctors calculated Mom's malignant tumor to be at stage IV. In plain English, that meant that the tumor was cancerous and it had spread to other organs. Furthermore, the results of the chest and abdomen CAT scan revealed lesions in the lungs and liver.

Then she reviewed the blood test. Surprisingly, the cancer marker was not very high. That meant that the progression of the disease did not match the blood test. At this point, my mom and I were just listening. A lot of the doctor's explanation was somewhat clear, but my mind was still so hazy from the previous experience that, as hard as I tried, I still could not absorb everything the doctor relayed. After Dr. Poplin finished going over all of the test results, I asked her who the doctor was that broke the news to us so abruptly. She looked at me with a look of surprise, but without emotion said that he was a doctor in training. We did not discuss that subject any further right then, but she later apologized telling us that they had a talk with the doctor in training. I also found out that she heard from the nurses how hard we took the news and how the pale color of our faces concerned them enough that they were ready to take both of us to the ER.

The next part of our conversation was about treatment options. There were only a few so it did not take too long to discuss them. The options were chemotherapy, radiation, pain management, and, if possible, surgery. Dr. Poplin explained that chemotherapy was an intravenous treatment that destroys cancer cells by stopping their ability to grow and divide. Radiation therapy used high-energy wave particles to destroy or damage cancer cells. Pain management was not a treatment, but if a patient experienced severe pain, the doctors would create a regimen that would help control the pain. Surgery was an option, but chemotherapy would have to follow to eliminate cancer cells and prevent recurrence. She said that both chemotherapy and radiation had the same success rate.

When I asked the doctor about the survival rate and specifications, she asked the nurse behind the desk to give me an information sheet. When I saw it, I was shocked. The information sheet listed the treatments, the side effects, percentages of success rates, and the length of time that each treatment prolongs life.

As I looked at the sheet and explained it to my mom, both of us were thinking of my aunt who passed away from ovarian cancer just a couple of months before. It brought back memories of what a poor quality of life she had during the last months of her life. She received chemotherapy treatment, which made her miserable. She was nauseous, and couldn't really eat anything without throwing up. She could not do much during the day because she had no strength to keep up and, frankly, no desire. She lost hair on her head and was depressed. She had many children and grandchildren that visited her at home many times a day. The visits definitely helped to get her mind off the sickness, but at the same time, she felt so sick that it really didn't matter. Later on, the pain was unbearable and the doctor prescribed very strong pain medication. Once that started, she wasn't mentally there. She slept most of the day not knowing when people came to visit. The times she was awake, she was very incoherent. From the time doctors diagnosed her to the end of her life, she lived three very long, painful, and practically nonexistent months.

As conversation arose regarding my aunt, we compared the treatment options on the list. According to the facts, the survival rate was only up to 4% with chemotherapy or radiation, and each extended life for only a month. Being that pancreatic cancer was deemed to be the most dreadful and most aggressive of all cancers, the survival rate was very low and it extended life for only one more month. That's it…only one month! It seems like a big price to pay for a person already suffering from this disease to add more misery, pain, hair loss, and other chemotherapy and radiation side effects simply to extend life for one more month. Of course, if there would be no more added pain and suffering and a good quality of life was factored in, then one more month of life extension would be wonderful. I would give anything for my mom to live just a little longer. I think anyone would. Wouldn't you?

My mom thought about it more, turned to me, and asked my opinion. I looked into her eyes searching for the answer she was looking for, but instead I saw anguish and confusion—a look that asked me for guidance. This chapter of our lives forced us to experience role reversal. I always looked to my mom to give me advice on many different issues no matter how big or small: personal or family and kids, she always had the right non-judgmental answer. Mom could deliver words of wisdom that hit home and made me smile. This time it was my turn and it was a big decision. Who was I to decide what to do with her life? Obviously, I wanted her to live a long life.

According to the diagnosis, this disease did not leave much room for hope and the treatments didn't mean much—only a 4% survival rate. There was no way to know if my mom would fall into that small category. If she did, she would be a very lucky woman. If she didn't, then the pain, suffering, and all the other anguish would have been for nothing. What would you have done? These questions circled in my brain repeatedly.

Without hesitation, I took my mom's hand, looked her in the eyes again, and explained to her that I would guide and support her through this process with all the heart and strength I have. I would go over the treatments, side effects, and survival rates with her again and give her the options that were available. I would help her understand and give her my opinion, but I couldn't decide for her. The ultimate decision would have to be hers. I love my mom...don't get me wrong. I love her very much, but I believe that people should make their own substantial choices—especially when it comes down to the future of their own bodies, their own minds.

My mom squeezed my hand as if to motion that it was okay and not to stress over it too much, but I couldn't help it. She said that she would not want to go through so much suffering. Whatever fate was in store for her, she would want to go with dignity, with hair, and sound mind. (Those were the exact words! Yes...the hair was important.)

We notified the doctor that we would take the information sheet home and discuss the test results and therapies that were available with the family before making any decisions.

Chapter 4:

Search for the Unknown:

Are There Any Other Treatments Besides What the Doctor Knows?

That evening, I drove my mom home. It was a long and mind-racking ride. All of the day's nuances and the doctors' words continued to haunt me. I was overwhelmed with emotions. I think that for me the news was still a shock and I was finally beginning to digest what had transpired that day. I could not believe my mom received a death sentence. She only had three months to live…I can't even say she had three months to enjoy her life. Just thinking about it made me cry. But no, I couldn't. I had to stop myself, afraid that she would wake up. I was afraid to make her upset and add to the stressful day. I quickly wiped the tears from my face and looked at Mom in the passenger seat. She was reclined and sleeping peacefully right next to me. I wish there was an easier way to tell my father and my brothers about what happened that day. They only knew that we spent a couple of hours at the CINJ—that was it. I told them that we would fill them in about everything that evening at my parent's house. I was not looking forward to reliving this day, but I had no choice in the matter.

When we walked into the house, I noticed that the table was set for what I guessed to be dinner. I did not eat anything all day, just drank water. I just couldn't. As my father escorted my mom into the hallway, she looked at him as tears poured out of her and started to hit him on the shoulders and screaming something that sounded like, "That's it, only three months left! I am dying! I will be dead in three months!" (My parents speak in Russian to each other so it sounded very dramatic…and it was!)

My father kissed her and hugged her. He walked her to the living room to sit with her on the sofa and they sobbed as he held her in his arms. I didn't know what really happened, but I dropped everything on the floor and just walked mechanically like a robot to the living room, hugged them both, and cried. I'm not sure how long we stayed in a group hug and cried, but the doorbell brought us back to reality. The bell rang again. We stopped crying and all just stared at the door. It rang again. I finally realized that it was the doorbell.

My brothers walked in after I ran to open the door. They looked at me and saw my puffy red eyes. Without a word, they walked into the living room, sat next to my mom, and started sobbing. After a few minutes, I brought everyone some hot tea and tissues and asked that we compose ourselves to discuss the important information we received from the doctor's visit.

My mom and I told my father and brothers everything that happened that day including information regarding all the test results, diagnosis, and treatment options. We were all in agreement that chemotherapy and radiation treatments were not an option due to both the small percentage of survival rate and the numerous side effects that follow the treatment. We discussed surgery as a possibility depending on the success rate and viability. We needed to get recommendations of a good surgeon and make an appointment soon. We didn't know what else to do. We did not know much about the disease, except for the fact that it kills people with a lot of physical and mental suffering during the process. We knew that we only had the next three months to spend with Mom according to the doctor and the statistics.

After spending about three hours at my parents' house, I finally went home to my family. It was a long drive home after a long and emotionally stressful day. While driving, I was thinking about the next step and what my brothers and I should be doing in order to get Mom back on track. What exactly was it that we were dealing with? Did my mom really have incurable cancer? What is cancer altogether? Was traditional western medicine the only possible treatment available? Many questions surfaced and I did not have an answer for any of them. I knew that in order for me to get answers, I would have to learn all about the sickness first, and then about possible treatments if they existed. I also knew that I did not have a lot of time to do all of this. Every minute, hour, and day was precious.

I spent the next week piecing together information from various research angles to learn everything I could about cancer. My research began by searching the Internet. I watched numerous informative videos. I read books and articles that pertained to health and cancer. I can't say that all the information was useful, but I learned a little from everything I read and watched. I discovered that supplements that can help suppress cancer growth. I found other possible treatments, but these were not part of the conventional medicine world, so insurance did not cover them. It was clear that out of pocket expenses were inevitable if we were to go that route. I was amazed at all the information that was available and shared it with my mom, my father, and my brothers.

What exactly is cancer?

This was the first question I wanted to answer. Before we even get to that, we have to understand that our bodies are made of trillions of living cells, which have different functions. Normal body cells grow and divide in order to make new cells and then die in an orderly way. In the early years of a person's life, normal cells divide faster in order to allow the person to grow. After the person becomes an adult, most cells divide only to replace worn out or dying cells, or to repair an injury.

Cancer is the uncontrolled growth of abnormal cells in the body. Cancer starts when cells in a part of the body grow out of control. Cancer cell growth is different from normal cell growth in that, instead of dying, cancer cells continue to reproduce and form new abnormal cells. Cancer cells can invade adjacent organs and spread to other tissues, which can be life threatening. Normal cells do not do that. A cell that grows out of control and invades other tissues is what specifies a cell to be a cancer cell. The extra abnormal cells that have multiplied form a mass of tissue called a tumor—specifically, a malignant tumor. Over time, the tumors can replace normal tissue, crowd it, or push it aside.[2]

"Unbelievable," I thought. Your body loses control of the normal function and abnormal cells take over—sort of like an alien invasion. Now that I understood what cancer was, I was ready to find the answer to my next question.

How and why does a normal cell become a cancer cell?

Cells become cancer cells because of damaged deoxyribonucleic acid (DNA) molecules. Imagine that every cell has DNA inside it and it contains a set of instructions telling the cell how to grow and divide. Now imagine that the set of instructions modify (mutate) and contain errors. Those errors allow a cell to become cancerous. A couple of things can happen if there is a mutation. For one, mutated cell DNA can instruct a healthy cell to grow and divide more rapidly by creating new cells with the same mutation. Another possibility that leads to cancer is when a cell recognizes an error in the DNA instructions, but unsuccessfully tries to repair itself by making corrections.[3]

Okay, so how did we get here? What causes these mutations or changes to our cells? There are a couple of reasons changes occur. Sometimes we can inherit mutations from our parents, which account for a very small percentage. Generally, though, DNA damage is either the result of cell reproduction errors or influences from the environment. Examples of environmental influences are smoking, radiation, viruses, obesity, hormones, chronic inflammation, and lack of exercise. Wow! We can probably prevent most of the reasons just mentioned. But who thinks about them as you are going through life?

Sometimes we are so busy that we don't even stop to look at ourselves to think about what we can do to make ourselves healthier. There is no time—or so we say. We make excuses every day thinking we are not strong enough to make certain changes in our lives. Everyone has to make time now—not tomorrow, not next week, and not next month..........NOW. You need to take preventative measures now so that cancer does not creep into your life. When it is too late, you will realize that you should have, could have, and would have done something about it before.

What is a malignant tumor?
When cells multiply uncontrollably due to DNA damage and now all newly forming cells are cancerous, a mass can grow. We call this growth a malignant tumor or cancer.

If the cancer has grown in one organ, how does it spread to other organs?
How is it that cancer can get from the brain, let's say, to the liver? In my mom's case, how could it spread from the pancreas to the liver and lungs? Cancer proliferation is a very interesting but complicated process. I read about proliferation many times until I understood it clearly. It was very important for me to understand what cancer is, how it spreads, and how it survives in order to select the proper treatments that are available. Without having an understanding about the disease and what makes it live or die, I was afraid that I

would choose the wrong treatment—a treatment that would not help my mom.

I tried to explain my research in the simplest words I could to my mom, dad, and brothers. First, I relayed a couple of facts about the spreading of cancer. When cancer spreads, it is called metastatic cancer. Metastatic cancer can spread from the place it first started to another location in the body. It has the same name and the same type of cancer cells as the original cancer. The most common sites of cancer metastasis are the bones, liver, and lungs.

My mom's CAT scan showed lesions in the liver and the lungs. Based on my research, it made sense that the scan revealed metastasis.

More about the spreading (metastasis) of cancer

Cancer cells travel to other parts of the body when they get into the body's bloodstream or lymph vessels. If the cancer cells go into small blood vessels, they can get into the blood stream. The circulating blood sweeps cancer cells along until they affix somewhere. Usually they get stuck in a capillary, which is a very small blood vessel. Then the cells move through the wall of the capillary and into the tissue of a nearby organ. The cell can multiply to form a new tumor if the conditions are right for it to grow and it has the nutrients that it needs. This is a complicated process, which most cancer cells do not survive. Out of many thousands of cancer cells that reach the blood circulation, probably only a few will survive to form a secondary cancer, or metastasis.

During the process, white blood cells in our immune system may destroy some cancer cells. Sometimes fast flowing blood batters and eliminates cancer cells. To protect themselves, circulating cancer cells may try to stick to platelets to form clumps. Platelets are blood cells that help the blood to clot. Clinging to platelets can help cancer cells filter into upcoming capillary networks. This process can guide mutated cells to find a home in surrounding tissues.

Another way cancer cells travel to other parts of the body is through the lymphatic system. The lymphatic system is a network of tubes and glands that filters body fluid and fights infection. It also traps damaged or harmful cells such as cancer cells. If cancer cells go into the small lymph vessels close to the primary tumor, they can lodge into nearby lymph glands (technically known as nodes). Once affixed, the node may destroy the cancer cells, but some cells survive and grow to form tumors in one or more lymph nodes. When that happens, doctors may say that the cancer has spread to lymph nodes.

Cancer spreads in one last way: ***angiogenesis***, which is the formation of new blood vessels. Cancers use this process in order to increase the blood supply to the tumor. The tumor cannot grow beyond the size of a pinhead (1 to 2 mm) by itself. It needs to form new blood vessels to obtain a blood supply. The tumor's growth depends on the continued obtaining of necessary oxygen and nutrients from the blood supply.[4, 5]

Finding this information was fascinating! All I needed to do was find something that stopped angiogenesis, which would kill off the blood supply to the tumor and the tumor would stop growing. I know that it was not going to be that simple, but you never know. The next step was to research the stages of cancers and what they mean.

What are the four stages of cancer?

I researched pancreatic cancer staging in particular. The reason staging is necessary is because the doctors want to know how far the disease has progressed and what treatment options would work best. Cancer stages I through IV are categorized as such to reveal the cancer's progress based on the results of exams, imaging tests, and biopsies. Based on my mom's tests, she was stage IV, the most advanced stage. I will list and explain the other stages, just so that you can understand the difference between them.

Stage I – The tumor is confined to the pancreas and can be smaller or larger than 2 cm. It has not spread to nearby lymph nodes or other distant organs.

Stage II – The tumor is either confined to the pancreas or growing outside the pancreas but not into major blood vessels or nerves. It has not spread to nearby lymph nodes or other distant organs.

Stage III – The tumor is growing outside the pancreas into nearby major blood vessels or nerves. It may or may have not spread to nearby lymph nodes, and it has not spread to other distant organs.

Stage IV – The cancer has spread to distant lymph nodes or to distant organs. This is the most advanced and last stage that exists.[6]

As I read the information about the stages of cancer, I realized that my mom's diagnosis revealed something advanced. Stage IV—cancer spread to lymph nodes or possibly other organs. Doctors didn't mention lymph nodes, but they did mention *other organs*. This was not a possibility. It was reality. It was a fact that she had lesions in the liver and the lung, which can grow into cancer. Because it was a lesion and no biopsy was performed to confirm it was cancer, it could not be called cancer.

The oncologist urged us to see a ***pulmonologist***, a lung doctor. The oncologist also strongly recommended doing a biopsy. After finding out about the procedure and what was involved, there was no way my mom or I would agree to do it. Having gone through a biopsy of the pancreas, knowing it was not an easy procedure, and recognizing the state my mom was in, I did not want to aggravate her and see her suffer any further. Besides, I wanted to concentrate on her pancreas at that time.

I remembered reading an article about cutting off the blood supply to distant tumors to force the cancer to concentrate on growing and supplying the main tumor with nutrients. So, I thought if I concentrated on the main tumor, I would be doing the right thing. Were the doctors right in telling me that Mom only had three months to live? I did not want to believe it.

Day and night, I searched for the unknown. I made appointments to numerous doctors, specialists, and surgeons. Repeatedly, I heard the same response, "There is no real cure." The only offers were chemotherapy, radiation treatments, or surgery. Chemotherapy and radiation treatments came with a very small percentage of survival and really tough side effects like nausea and vomiting, hair loss, anemia, fatigue, infections, bleeding problems, skin and nail changes, memory changes, and the list goes on.

You might ask, "Why all the side effects?" Treatments of toxic drugs or rays of radiation affect both cancerous and normal cells. Both normal and cancer cells die, which creates organ functionality problems, which creates other side effects. It was not an option for my mom to take on this treatment knowing that her life span would only increase by one month while dealing with the daily side effects.

After having long conversations, we decided that the pain and side effects did not make life worth living. My mom said to me, "Let me die with dignity. I want to live whatever time I have left without added pain and suffering. I want my hair to be on my head and my skin to be intact. I want to spend quality time with my husband, my kids, and my grand kids." We would cry very often not knowing if the next day would be her last.

Of all the appointments to specialists and surgeons, two visits presented interest and stuck in my mind. One was the visit to a general surgeon in Brooklyn. It was a beautiful day and the weather was perfect—warm with a breeze coming from the ocean. We arrived early since there was no traffic and decided to take a stroll in a nearby park. With my help, we walked slowly through the park enjoying the nature around us. The beautiful trees and planted flowers were well-kept homes for the chirping birds flying about happily. We really took all of G-d's creations seriously and talked about the gift of life that we get while on this earth. Knowing that your life may be at the end makes you appreciate everything and not take it for granted.

Carrying the big envelopes containing films of CAT scans and other X-rays, we walked up to the surgeon's office on the second floor. We didn't wait long and were escorted into an office room where the surgeon was waiting. He greeted us courteously and told us to sit down. I gave him the X-rays, which he laid down on the table. I explained that we were possibly thinking of doing surgery to remove the cancer and wanted to know the procedure and success rate. The surgeon explained that the procedure was simple and that he would make an incision, cut out the tumor, suture it back up, and my mom would be all better. He further explained that since the tumor was at the tail of the pancreas and not in the heart of the pancreas, it was less involved and would be an easy procedure.

I looked at him and wondered why he was painting such a pretty picture. It sounded fairly simple and successful, but for some reason I was still skeptical. After seeing other doctors and hearing the prognosis of all treatments, this just did not make sense. I asked him about the healing process and success he had with other cancer patients, in particular pancreatic cancer. He looked at me and said, "Don't worry everything will be alright. After surgery, you will not have cancer. You will not have any more pain."

As my mom and I looked at each other and paid close attention to every word, my mind was racing. I looked around and saw the films still on the table. He didn't even look at the X-rays and CAT films before telling us that everything would be alright! I asked if he could look at the films. His response was, "That will not be necessary. I have years of experience and I am sure I will not see anything different than I already have in the past."

I wondered how he could have given us a response and tell us that my mom would be a great candidate for surgery if he didn't even look at the films? Everywhere else I took Mom, the first thing they did was look at the films to see what they are dealing with. I guessed the surgeon was a genius and saw straight through the envelope or he was overly confident in his skills to be able to make that kind of judgment in five minutes without looking at the films. I wanted to give him the benefit and think positive, but he did not sound very convincing. It was strange that he didn't do a physical exam, nor did he ask any questions regarding mom's health history, her up-to-date test results, or any other relevant information. He told us that surgery was imperative as soon as possible. Furthermore, he informed us that he was available to do the surgery as early as next week.

We thanked him for his time and said that we needed to think and talk to the family before making a decision. Exiting the office, my mom asked me to take her back to the park to spend a little more time together before driving her home. She looked very peaceful as we walked in the park. I asked her what she was thinking as we walked. Her answer to me was very simple, "Don't worry. Everything will be alright." I didn't know whether to laugh or cry, but I broke out with laughter knowing that her mind was made up about the surgery—at least with that surgeon.

The second interesting visit was to an oncology practice where the doctor combined traditional chemotherapy methods with alternative treatments that aimed at alleviating side effects. I thought it would be good to go for a second opinion and to see what additional treatments this practice offered. When I called for some information about the other treatments, the person taking the call did not offer details, but rather, told me that I needed to make an appointment.

I gave mom's info to a girl at the reception when we walked in and then sat down to wait. There were many others waiting in the reception to see the doctor. Most looked deathly ill. Some were skinny and appeared to have no hair under a head covering. Some had black and blue arms, which I guessed an IV caused. They all had something in common. They were all unhappy. No one wore a smile and the room's tension was thick. In total, we waited for about an hour and a half with me going to the reception about half way through to discover that the doctor only took new patients once he freed up. Fifteen minutes later, we were sitting in the doctor's office.

The doctor greeted us and we sat down in the chairs. She seemed preoccupied as she had many patients waiting for her. We spoke to her for five minutes explaining our situation. I asked about the other treatment she offered to her patients. The doctor cut me short and told me that the other treatments were IV infusions to help cancer patients ease the side effects. I thought this sounded great! I asked her if she could do these IV infusions without administering chemotherapy. "Absolutely not," she replied!

All of a sudden, she got up from her seat, said we were wasting her time, and left the room. Mom and I looked at each other and thought the doctor's actions were a little rude. I was simply trying to find the missing information I could not get over the phone. I wanted to know if this practice offered other treatments besides chemotherapy. Instead, after waiting all that time to see a doctor, I discovered that the other treatment was only available if you do chemotherapy. The doctor didn't want to hear that my mom wasn't interested in receiving chemotherapy.

I believed there was a reason for everything that happened. I had to come to this practice to learn that other forms of treatment existed. That information opened the door to many other possibilities, as you will see.

Chapter 5:

Alternative Treatments

IV Infusions and Supplements

As my search continued for the unknown, I thought that other people must be just as hungry for the same kind of information. There was another world out there, the world that the Food and Drug Administration (FDA) did not regulate. The FDA is a federal agency that is responsible for protecting public health by regulating and supervising food safety, dietary supplements, prescriptions, and many other categories. This agency gives its stamp of approval for medication and treatments that have gone through the necessary trials. The concept is good, but I discovered that many non-regulated FDA supplements that are natural and made from different plants, roots of plants, fruits, vegetables, and other natural substances are not deemed safe by many people.

My brother purchased a book called *Sharks Don't Get Cancer,* by William I. Lane and Linda Comac. After reading the book, he was convinced Mom should take **shark cartilage**—one of the supplements that the FDA did not regulate. Years of research led several doctors to make claims that they proved shark cartilage contained a protein that inhibited the formation of blood vessels to tumors. If a tumor could not create a blood vessel network, it would become malnourished and eventually die. Furthermore, the doctors claimed, if used properly, shark cartilage could prevent the development of tumor-based cancer and metastasis—stopping tumor growth. This claim was very powerful and promising. We wanted to know what specifically made shark cartilage (and not any other cartilage) so great.

We discovered that sharks, unlike other animals, have skeletons largely made up of cartilage, which is a tough yet malleable connective tissue. Amazingly, cartilage is a tissue that performs its functions without nerves, blood vessels, or a lymphatic system, and, therefore, blood does not transport nutrients to the cartilage. Known as amazing living machines, sharks rarely develop cancer. They have survived literally unchanged despite the fact that almost all other creatures of land and sea regularly incur cancer.

My brother shared this information with my mom and the rest of the family, and Mom decided to try it. There were no other promising options, and if this worked, it would be great! He discovered that supplement stores offered shark cartilage in either a powdered or a liquid form, which people could take orally or rectally. Since Mom had issues with taking meds orally, and to spare her any more pain, he ordered the powder form. The research claimed that when taken regularly, this treatment supposedly not only inhibits angiogenesis as stated before, but also stimulates the immune system, which then works synergistically with the protein in fighting disease.

Another supplement that we thought was important for my mom to take was ***milk thistle***. The most important reason was because she had a lesion in her liver and we were very worried that it would grow into cancer. We wanted her to have protection. Remember, the liver is a very large organ and it has many functions. People make medicine from milk thistle's above ground seeds and plant parts. It is a gentle supplement mostly used for liver disorders. It protects cells from toxic chemicals and drugs, and has antioxidant and anti-inflammatory effects. I purchased it for Mom and she took it every day.

I was happy that we found shark cartilage and milk thistle for my mom, but these were not enough. I wanted to do more. I read on an Internet site that it was very important to build up your immune system if you wanted to get healthy and fight disease. I had to find something else to boost my mom's immune system. There were many supplements, but I didn't have the luxury of time to try them out on her to see which one works best. Besides, I didn't want her to take many pills because of the complaints she had every time she ate something. Don't get me wrong, it's not that I minded talking to her many hours a day and asking her how she felt at certain times of the day, it's just that I didn't want her to have unnecessary pain.

After thinking a long while, I remembered the oncologist we visited offering *other treatments* to her patients who elected to receive chemotherapy. I remembered her saying something about giving patients vitamin IVs. I searched the Internet for possibilities and plugged in different words to find something. After a long search, I found a wellness center that piqued my interest. The center was in Mount Kisco and went by the name Advanced Medicine of Mt. Kisco. (That was the name at that time. Now the center is in a different location and goes by the Integrated Medicine of Mount Kisco.) They had both a medical doctor and a doctor of nutrition on staff. I called and made the next available appointment for a consultation hoping my mom would later give her blessing.

We waited three days for our appointment and then we were on our way. I picked up my mom from her home and drove her to Mount Kisco (a town in Westchester). It was a pretty area.

I parked and helped my mom out of the car. She was very frail. On top of the pancreatic cancer, she had acquired diabetes. It was very common since the pancreas lost function of making insulin due to the cancer. Mom was on diabetes medication, but was in the beginning stages, so we were still trying to figure out if the dosage was good since her diet was not the best. If she ate a full meal, she was ok—but when she ate very little, her blood sugar would be low and she would not feel well at all.

We walked to the building and Mom had to rest a little. Climbing the couple of steps, I could see that she was weak and hesitating. I came closer, put my hand under her arm and helped her walk up the stairs. You have to understand that my mom didn't weigh so little and I was petite, so it was hard for me to lift her weight up the stairs with the bags that I had on my shoulder. As we walked up the last step, I felt like the weight was getting heavier. I looked at Mom's face and saw her slightly fainting.

I quickly opened the door to the office and screamed, "HELP!" I was afraid I was not going to be able to support Mom and she was going to fall down the stairs. I was petrified. My knees were shaking. A gentleman ran to the door and helped me carry Mom inside, then helped her sit in a chair. Mom was going in and out of consciousness. She kept on saying to me, "Don't be scared. I am ok." I quickly gave her a candy that she learned to carry with her after searching her pockets. Her blood sugar must have been low. After she had two candies and some water she was much better. I held her hand the whole time. I loved her so much and didn't want to lose her.

When our time arrived, a receptionist greeted and escorted us to an office where we met with the Doctor of Nutrition, Michael Wald. He was very courteous and warm as he introduced himself. As he spoke to us, my mom and I knew we were in the right place. He told us that he had multiple sclerosis and was trying to cure himself naturally because there was no real cure in western medicine.

After going over Mom's health history extensively, he had us meet with the MD who also looked over the health history document. He asked us additional questions and suggested we do a Darkfield Exam, which would tell him exactly what was going on with Mom's blood. The MD would use the results to reveal a path so he could suggest a protocol. A Darkfield Exam consisted of putting a drop of blood on a slide and looking at it under the microscope—a blood analysis test. He was able to see red blood cells, white blood cells, platelets, and other activity in the blood. Even though we did not see it ourselves, we thought it was a unique process.

After he looked at the slide, he had a machine print a very long report. The report listed vitamin and mineral deficiencies. This information was amazing—the doctor completed a very real and informative test. Michael Wald explained that a person is likely to get sick with a compromised immune system. The immune system protects us from any foreign substance that enters our body by fighting and getting rid of the substance. Sometimes it fails when a germ successfully invades, which makes you sick. With cancer, the cells may produce signals that reduce the immune system's ability to detect and kill tumor cells, or they may have changes that make it harder for the immune system to recognize and target them. Because of the compromised communication, cancer can develop and go unnoticed for many years until symptoms arise.

At the end of the consultation, Michael Wald gave Mom a couple of supplements that were supposed to alleviate her pain naturally. He also suggested doing some IV treatments—vitamin and mineral IV infusion into the vein to be absorbed right away, without the body needing to process it. The intention was for my mom's immune system to grow stronger and receive a boost from the IV supplements, which could give her an appetite and help her with the pain.

This sounded too good to be true. I had to stay positive and believe that we came to this place for a reason. Michael Wald was very knowledgeable and very believable. It was definitely a very interesting approach. Not only was it an interesting approach, but a very expensive one as well. I couldn't think about the cost at that particular moment and concentrated on making my mom well.

The protocol consisted of IV infusions twice a week and a regimen of supplements. My mom agreed to the protocol at least for now to see how she would be feeling. The next step was to come back for a follow-up appointment two weeks later to check on her progress and decide if any protocol changes were necessary.

We went home that afternoon feeling uplifted thanks to the wellness center and Michael Wald. I felt that his approach was a very good one. What he was doing was amazing: getting to the root of the problem and treating symptoms rather than masking them.

Although my mom's case was very different and she had an advanced stage of cancer, I had optimism. I was not sure if this treatment would cure her, but was hoping it would help her gain back physical strength and improve her state of mind. My mom's intellect was still sharp, but she was very depressed wondering if every day was her last. She knew that she was dying. After all, she only had three months to live. She always had that thought in the back of her mind and often spoke about it.

We paid a visit to Dr. Poplin, the oncologist at CINJ. At that time, Mom underwent two weeks of IV treatments and one month of shark cartilage and milk thistle. She was feeling a little stronger and had less pain than the last time she was at CINJ. Since the shark cartilage was administered rectally, Mom was concerned about the doctor noticing the white residue. She asked me what she should say to Dr. Poplin regarding her current treatments. My mom was worried that the doctor would not approve with what she was doing. I told her not to worry and just be honest.

Dr. Poplin did a full physical exam including carefully checking her extremities. She said that everything was still the same as last time. She asked Mom about how she was feeling and if there are any changes in the severity of pain. She also asked if Mom was on any type of treatment. Mom looked at me; I gave her a nod of approval and then at the doctor. She told the doctor that she was taking supplements and doing vitamin IVs. The doctor didn't say much about it nor was there any negative or positive remarks. She just noted it in the chart. After doing a rectal exam, she asked about the white stuff that looked like chalk. I explained that Mom used shark cartilage enemas with the hope of helping with the disease. The doctor did not comment except for asking Mom to be careful. The doctor assigned a blood test with special cancer markers and other important factors that were relevant to Mom's sickness.

When we heard from the doctor regarding the blood results a couple of days later, she informed us that there was no change from the last blood test. Everything was status quo. I felt that no change was a good thing. As long as all the major organs continued functioning according to the blood test, I was happy. My mom continued taking the supplements while going to the wellness center for treatment.

During that time, I continued my search for other alternative treatments and anything else I could discover regarding cancer. I found and read many books about healing the body and building the immune system. Two books I highly recommend are *Spontaneous Healing* and *Natural Health, Natural Healing,* both by Dr. Weil, who I absolutely adore and believe in. The books really resonated with me—especially what he was trying to teach me about how our bodies work and heal. I was amazed to read that the human body, given the chance, can heal by itself.

Continuing the online search, I stumbled upon a procedure called **body radiosurgery,** which is a type of radiation treatment. It was not the same as the traditional radiation treatment doctors offered my mom. It seemed that it was not a very popular procedure. In fact, it was an innovative treatment. At that time, the special machines that administered body radiosurgery were only available in three countries: Japan, England, and the United States. I was very eager to find more information about this process.

I called to request information and they said that they would send me a VHS tape offering all the information about the procedure. I was waiting for this tape like there was no tomorrow. A couple of days later, I received and watched the tape immediately. I had to watch it three times to understand and digest all of the information. It blew me away—I was speechless. Why was no one talking about this procedure? Before telling you what amazed me about the tape, I'm going to define body radiosurgery using a pamphlet from found online. Gil Lederman summarizes the same sentiment from the video on his pamphlet:

> The principle of Body Radiosurgery is precise non-invasive delivery of high radiation doses to the cancer while normal healthy surrounding tissues are, in general, spared the effects of the radiation beam. This is in marked contrast to standard radiation, which is much less able to protect normal tissues from radiation effects. (p. 10)

Now I'll explain what I remember from the tape. The video narrator started by explaining the concept of body radiosurgery. He said that body radiosurgery is neither invasive nor surgery. The following is a paraphrased continuation of the information from the video: a patient can use this procedure to treat primary and metastatic tumors. Compared to standard external beam radiation, a doctor can administer higher radiation doses with potentially fewer treatments while yielding superior results. It is likely that radiosurgery will control many cancers resistant to standard radiation. The usage of the word *control* in the previous sentence does not necessarily mean *cure*. It means that the cancer in the treated area stops growing, shrinks, or disappears. This method treats a long list of cancers including pancreatic cancer.

As I watched the video, I was looking for one piece of very important information. I wanted to know the success rate based on experience with this procedure. At the end of the tape, the narrator mentioned that the procedure was 90% successful. I rewound it many times to make sure I was hearing that statement correctly. Could this be true—not 2%, not 4%, but 90%? This was crazy! I was astonished at what I heard—happy, but none the less astonished. Tears were rolling down my cheeks from joy knowing that this procedure could potentially give my mom a longer life. I could not believe that something like this existed, but not spoken about by doctors. The difference between success rates was huge. It was life versus death. I thought I was so lucky to have found this information. I was so eager to share this information with my mom and the rest of the family. I was sure everyone would be just as happy as I was.

A question kept circling in my mind: why were the general public doctors we saw not talking about this procedure? How could professional medical oncologists live with themselves after telling a patient that they have only a couple months to live and not offer treatment options other than traditional radiation and chemotherapy knowing that the success rate is so low and will not give their patients a good quality of remaining life in this world? If doctors put other options on the table, they may save and spare many more lives from suffering. I don't know the answers to these questions. Maybe they just don't know. Maybe they know and don't believe in these treatments. Maybe they don't have time to learn about other possible treatments that exist. I did not have a good answer for these questions.

Chapter 6:

Innovative Treatment

Body Radiosurgery

The next step was to call and set everything up. The woman who answered the phone informed me that the machine for body radiosurgery was in Staten Island University Hospital and the program was lead by Dr. Gil Lederman. Wow! That was not far at all. I was willing to take my mom to another state—no matter what the distance would have been—but this was even better.

The woman mentioned that we had to go through a process before visiting for an initial appointment. First, we had to send mom's CAT scans, blood work, and other imaging to the hospital for Dr. Lederman to review. After Dr. Lederman analyzed all the information and decided that Mom could be a candidate for this procedure, then he would review mom's case with a panel of doctors on his staff. At this peer review, the doctors present a patient's case, review all tests, and decide whether he or she may be a candidate for this procedure. At that point, they would call to let us know what the next steps were if Mom was a candidate.

It was nerve racking to know that my mom might not be a candidate for this procedure. Now that I found something that had such a high success rate and seemed to be a very promising procedure, I was very persistent to push the chances of her candidacy and move the process along. I so hoped that they would consider her.

As I listened carefully, my sense of purpose intensified. I needed to make sure Dr. Lederman had all of Mom's necessary tests and films as soon as possible. It took me two days of coordinating with my family to deliver all the CAT scans and blood tests to Staten Island University Hospital. My mom's main documentation included the ER scan, and both the CINJ and primary doctor information.

My family was ecstatic about the procedure, especially my mom who couldn't stop hugging and kissing me—but we still had to wait for the answer. While patiently waiting, I noticed a change in mom's outlook on life. It looked like she had hope shining on her face. She had a more positive attitude when we spoke and was a little happier. As a family, we were glad to see such an important transformation before our eyes. She was still very sick and in pain, but it was a nice change of pace to see her smiling from time to time. The mind is so powerful. Your emotions really can bring you down or lift you up.

About a week and a half later, I got a call from a nurse on Dr. Lederman's staff. She informed me that the doctors reviewed my mom's case and the team decided that she was a candidate for this procedure. I screamed with joy, "Yes! Thank you! Thank you so much!" I didn't realize that people were around me and I was speaking very loudly. I was so happy that my mom was approved for this procedure and couldn't contain how lucky she and our whole family was. Perhaps my happiness was premature, but I was excited to know that there was a treatment with a high success rate and my mom had a shot at it. The nurse scheduled an initial consultation with Dr. Lederman.

That evening, I headed straight for Queens. I ran into my parents' house, found my mom and gave her a big hug and a kiss. I slowly told her that she was approved for the procedure at Staten Island University Hospital.

I think I was happier than she was. Maybe she just didn't know what to expect? Or didn't want to get her hopes up? She was very melancholy. She said that the physical pain she underwent every time she ate gave her no hope of beating a disease that no one survived. I tried to comfort her and get her hopes up a little. I explained that Dr. Lederman had a team of doctors look at her films and other tests. They made a decision that she would be a candidate for the procedure. If a bunch of doctors thought that she had a chance to survive, maybe she should do the same.

"Think positive Mama!" I said, "We should be grateful for the chance to have this treatment. Who knows, maybe it will make you feel better. We have to hope for the best." After some time, the sadness broke and I could see a little smile.

I drove my mom to Staten Island University Hospital to see Dr. Lederman for the initial consultation. After entering the office, a receptionist asked for our name then told us to sit and wait with the others. As we walked to open seats, we stared unintentionally at the cancer patients waiting to be called. It was a scary sight. Some had swelling on their foreheads while others had something strangely wrong with their necks. I really felt bad for those people and hoped that they would get better soon. We found seats and patiently waited to be called.

Shortly after, a nurse escorted us to the doctor's office. Dr. Lederman was very polite, but shifted the conversation to business. He thoroughly went over mom's health history and up-to-date treatments. Then he went over his team's discussion that took place during the review process. According to all her completed tests, he said that Mom's results, including the size of the tumor, indicated that she was, indeed, a candidate for the procedure. He said he predominantly performed brain and neck tumor procedures for individuals. They had completed procedures for body tumors, but just not as often. He assured us not to worry, but said many people are skeptical because it is an innovative treatment.

Furthermore, he explained that the body tumors are receptive to the procedure and the success rate was relatively high. Based on mom's large tumor, she would probably need more than one treatment, each lasting approximately thirty minutes. The number of sessions would be decided upon preliminary testing.

Preparation for the procedure required completion of a couple of very important steps. Dr. Lederman explained that there would be many physicians on staff with different qualifications around Mom all the time and that we should not be alarmed. All of them would be working together.

A specialist would make a custom-fit body radiosurgery frame and conduct multiple quality assurance steps to ensure precision during the administering of the procedure. The frame was necessary to help hold Mom securely to focus the beam. Then a technician would take high-resolution CAT and MRI scans with Mom in the *fiducial*-marked stereotactic body frame. This provided a map to localize the cancer and perform body radiosurgery. Fiducial markers, which are located within the custom fit frame, helped the staff precisely guide the beam to its target. This process allowed cancer localization for computerized treatment planning.

At that time, they would decide the number of treatments. I asked Dr. Lederman what to expect during the procedure and if there would be any side effects. His response made me somewhat happy. He advised us there should be no pain or any discomfort during the procedure. She should not experience any major side effects except for fatigue—and even that would dissipate within days.

He was silent for a second and then mentioned one side effect that might affect Mom in an adverse way. Since there would be highly concentrated beams directed to the pancreas and they would have to go through the stomach, there might be a chance that an ulcer could develop because of the procedure. An ulcer was something to consider. I looked at my mom to see that she was a bit confused. I explained to Mom everything the doctor said and I could see her thinking hard.

She turned at that point and said, "Doctor, do you think this radiation would help me? I am so tired of this pain that I am having. I just want it to go away."

Dr. Lederman looked at my mom and said, "I can't guarantee that it will help you, but I know that it did help many people before you."

I explained to my mom that the doctor couldn't legally guarantee that the procedure would cure her simply because that's what she wanted to hear. I know I would want a guarantee if I were in her place. Wouldn't you?

After the doctor finished going over all the important information regarding the procedure, he wanted us to go home, relay everything to the family, and then make a group decision. He instructed us to call the office as soon as we knew our answer. We thanked him and went home.

That evening, my family gathered around the dinner table to discuss the plan of action regarding the Dr. Lederman procedure. Honestly, it was not such a hard decision. We all agreed that body radiosurgery would be the best choice for Mom at that time. The fact that the success rate was high and the only major side effect was, perhaps, getting an ulcer, really made our decision easy. If an ulcer did develop, we hoped it could quickly heal. My mom was very happy to move forward with the procedure, so I called the next day to make the appointment.

The journey of stereotactic body radiosurgery at Staten Island University Hospital felt like a lifetime of anticipation. We worried about the after effects, but trusted the decision would be rewarding. Dr. Lederman's explanation of everything Mom would experience was very accurate—all the steps he mentioned—getting a custom-fit mold built for Mom all the way through the actual procedure. My mom received five thirty-minute treatments in a span of two weeks. She was tired after the treatment, but did not have any other side effects.

During the two weeks Mom received treatment at Staten Island University Hospital, she still went for IVs twice a week, took supplements, and even visited the Cancer Institute of New Jersey for her scheduled appointment. The IV infusions really helped strengthen her immune system and she was able to tolerate the treatment better. When Mom went to CINJ for an appointment, the oncologist performed a comprehensive physical exam and was happy to see that Mom was not worse than before, nor the same as last time she saw her, but a little better.

We communicated with the oncologist about Mom's body radiosurgery procedures, but she had never heard of it and had no comment. We also let the doctor know that we were continuing with IVs and supplements. She did not ask about the supplements, but instead gave us a smile and said, "If you think it is helping you, then continue with it."

Chapter 7:

Revamping the Diet

As our search for answers on surviving cancer continued, we realized that food played a very big role in my mom's recovery process. Eating the way she did, even though she still lacked appetite, would not help her beat cancer. In order to understand my mom's food practices at that time, there is relevant information you should be aware of regarding her past diet.

Because my mom was one of eight children, it was very hard to provide food for her father and for such a big family. It was hard work, but they managed. The food was mostly simple, but satisfying. While she was growing up, her food consisted of white bread, butter, honey (that her older brother made in the backyard of his house), milk, and hot cereal like farina. They would also eat cold cuts, white potatoes, soups made from boiling beef bones or chicken bones with chick peas, beans and pasta, borsht (soup with cabbage, beets and carrots), and soup with meat balls. Sometimes they made fish soup, called *ucha,* where the fish was boiled for a very long time and then vegetables were added to make a hearty meal.

At least once a week they had festive dishes with rice and either beef, turkey, or vegetables. Most of the time a piece of finely cut beef fat was added to the rice dishes to make them soft and more flavorful. Fish was made as well, but there was no variety. Carp was a very popular choice and was always deep fried and served once a week and on special occasions. On those days, not only were fish and rice dishes made but also accompanied by a huge rack of veal roast or a whole boiled chicken. (This happened only if there was a big celebration like a wedding). Meat and fish were very expensive and not abundantly available, so they were only served once a week and on special occasions.

For dessert, a variety of nuts, seeds, and dried fruit were served. Examples of those would have been pistachios, walnuts, sunflower seeds, raisins, and dried apricots. Seasonal fruits and vegetables were available, but very expensive and most of the time grown on the trees in the back yard. For special occasions, simple pastries were made. Processed foods were almost nonexistent. Exceptions were made for special occasions when cake was served—and even then, it was a very expensive treat. As you can see, 99% of food was cooked and made at home. This was very economical and fed the whole family with the known ingredients.

I almost forgot to mention drinks. During and after a meal, people welcomed hot green or black tea even during the hot summer months. On special occasions and celebrations, they served vodka, home made beer and wine. In the summer, people enjoyed lemonade and homemade kvas, which is similar to barley malt.

When we came to the United States in 1979, the food frenzy definitely caught our eye. I remember going shopping to a supermarket with my mom for the first time. I will never forget that experience. We walked in and were amazed at the abundance of food. There were boxes and bags of the same thing with different labels. The filled shelves displayed many varieties of bread, cakes, pastries, potato chips, cereals I had never seen before, and many different colors of soda. What was all that stuff? All we knew was that it all looked good and we could not wait to sample some. What about all the baked goods? Twinkies, chocolate cupcakes with vanilla cream filling, ding dongs, little fruit pies, and all the donuts. We could not believe there were so many cakes and pastries—they all looked so delicious. Later, we did try many of them. My mom's favorite was a powdered donut.

Bread was one food item for which we could not acquire the taste. Out shopping for food, my parents bought Wonder Bread many times just to find out why people filled their carts with it. It was so soft and really had no taste. We were used to bread that had a taste and a very dense consistency, so my mom baked her own bread for many years. My mom used to say, "I can eat one piece of my baked bread and be satiated, but if I eat wonder bread, even after five slices I am still hungry!"

Fruits, vegetables, and even chicken and meat tasted different. Fruits and vegetables were definitely less flavorful and the color was not as rich. Meat and chicken had a different look to it and were much more fatty. My mom used to say, "I can cook a chicken here for half an hour and it will be done. Back home I had to cook chicken for more than an hour for it to be ready."

In Russia, my parents bought chicken and meat from a butcher. Usually, they bought what they were going to use that day or for the next two days. They never would have frozen meat or chicken to use later. Some relatives owned and raised their own chickens, sheep, and cow in their back yard and had fresh milk daily. Mom lived in the city, so she did not have her own chickens and cow.

As the years went by, slowly but surely we got used to the American diet. Our house always had soda and was the main drink at lunch and dinner. We ate donuts and many ready bought pastries for breakfast and even had them for snacks. The signature rice and meat dishes were still cooked and eaten regularly on weekends the same way as in Russia. Meat and chicken were consumed almost daily because of the abundance. Salads with different vegetables were enjoyed at every meal. We would regularly eat fruit as well. So all the dishes that Mom was used to eating in Russia were still made and consumed, but a lot of processed food and soda was added to the diet.

Diet is a very important factor for someone who has cancer. More than other diseases, cancer is a reflection of our modern environmental and lifestyle choices. The World Health Organization (WHO) publishes the World Cancer Report, which documents cancer trends, the frequency of cancer in different countries, and mortality rates. Their research suggests that approximately 4% of cancers are inherited or genetic; the rest are preventable and are linked to lifestyle, diet and the environment.[7]

It is imperative to look at what you are putting into your body and how it makes you feel. After all, what we eat becomes part of us. First, we chew our food, then it goes into our stomach to be digested. After food digests, it gets absorbed into our blood. Our blood is what creates our cells, our tissues, and our organs. Therefore, our food does not only affect our body, but it affects our thoughts and our minds, as well as how we are able to do the work that we enjoy and how we relate to people and our loved ones.[6]

For a person with cancer it is very important to cut out all the sugar from the diet. That means a very strict low to no simple sugar diet. It also means to avoid fruit at all expense. Sugar feeds cancer. I never understood why oncologists always have a tray of candy on the reception counter and offer it to their cancer patients after chemotherapy as they are leaving. I am sure the patient feels more energy right after eating the candy for a little while and then may feel a crash. This is a very interesting and important topic, but I will leave it for another book.

Cancer cells thrive on simple sugars. They cannot metabolize complex carbohydrates, fats, or proteins. When you starve cancer cells from sugar, they can't survive and ultimately die. It is also important to alkalize our bodies. What that means is that we have to eat foods that are alkaline like alkaline water, green powders that contain wheatgrass, barley grass, and algae. These substances alkalize the body. Cancer cells thrive in an acid environment and don't do well when the body is more alkaline.[8]

Let me explain cancer cell environment in a little more detail, because this was a very important factor in my mom's recovery. We as human beings are electrical beings just like all the other living organisms. Every healthy cell in a human body carries a measurable electromagnetic negative charge. Cells in an acidic, oxygen-deprived environment have an electromagnetic positive charge. Since the laws of electromagnetism demand that opposites attract, unhealthy cells and their acid attract and bind to healthy cells. This process increases the likelihood that healthy cells will be damaged by the acidic environment or by the cell fermentation process that occurs when inadequate oxygen is available for healthy cell function. When many of these damaged cells grow, they create a mass called a tumor.

As I explained in chapter 4, cancer cells can form from normal cells when DNA is modified as a result of any number of external factors, including radiation, chemicals and toxins, bacteria, viruses, fungi, parasites, and of course the water and food we ingest. If the immune system is not functioning properly or is overburdened, cancer cells can proliferate and effectively overpower its capacity to destroy them.

Many holistic experts considered cancer an effect of deep imbalance in the body, not a disease. These imbalances are caused by metabolic acids that build up in the blood and are released into cells, tissues, and organs. Food and water provide fuel for our bodies and feed us on the cellular level. If the fuel is excessively acidic, it builds an unhealthy cell environment, creating possibilities for mutations (DNA cell modifications). Acidity reduces oxygen, and cancer thrives in an oxygen poor and acid rich environment. Cancer cells can obtain energy through fermentation, a conversion process that does not require oxygen. While normal cells can no longer divide and survive in this type of acidic environment, cancer cells flourish even on the few available nutrients.

In 1931, Dr. Otto Warburg, one of the twentieth century's leading cell biologists, was awarded the Nobel Prize in Medicine for his research and action in metabolism of tumors and the respiration of cells, particularly cancer cells. Warburg's hypothesis, published in *The Prime Cause and Prevention of Cancer*, suggests that **anaerobiosis**, a process of energy production in a cell with no oxygen present, was a primary cause of cancerous cells. Dr. Warburg discovered that the root cause of cancer is too much acidity in the body, meaning that the pH, potential hydrogen, is below the normal level of 7.4, which constitutes an *acidic* state. He investigated the metabolism of tumors and the respiration of cells and discovered that cancer cells maintain and thrive in a lower pH, as low as 6.0, due to lactic acid production and elevated CO_2. He firmly believed that there was a direct relationship between pH and oxygen. Higher pH, which is alkaline, means higher concentration of oxygen molecules, while lower pH, which is acidic, means lower concentrations of oxygen.[11]

In his work *The Metabolism of Tumours,* Warburg demonstrated that all forms of cancer are characterized by two basic conditions: **acidosis** and **hypoxia** (lack of oxygen). Lack of oxygen and acidosis are two sides of the same coin: where you have one, you have the other. He further explained, "All normal cells have an absolute requirement for oxygen, but cancer cells can live without oxygen—a rule without exception. Deprive a cell 35% of its oxygen for 48 hours and it may become cancerous" (Warburg).

Let me explain why Warburg's hypothesis is relevant to my mom's and everyone else's health. Alkaline solutions generally absorb oxygen, while acidic solutions eject oxygen. By nature, our bodies' bodily fluids are alkaline with the exception of digestive juices and urine. In order to retain oxygen, our blood has to have a pH of approximately 7.4, an alkaline range. When the body lacks necessary minerals and nutrients, it becomes acidic. In order to maintain a pH of 7.4, the body turns on its natural mechanism to search for the missing minerals and nutrients from the organs. Since these organs are now missing the minerals and nutrients that it gave to the blood, the cells of these organs become acidic and their capability to take up oxygen-cell respiration is compromised. Deficiency in oxygen causes the cells to seek energy by converting glucose through fermentation. This produces more acid and lowers the pH even further. This process creates a perfect environment in which cancer cells can grow and multiply even though the body tries to correct the pH imbalance.

I cannot guarantee that a person can prevent cancer by reducing acid in his or her body, but at least there is a chance to cut off cancer cells from their means of survival. By changing the body's pH, the body heals itself by allowing it to function optimally, which destroys toxins including cancer cells before they accumulate. Cancer cells may exist even in a healthy body, but this scenario lends to the killing and removing of damaged cells before they grow and multiply to form a tumor.

In order to prepare Mom's body to fight cancer, it was very important to change her diet drastically. That meant that she had to cut out all the sugar and raise her pH level. It was easy to cut out most of the simple sugar from her diet, but getting rid of fruits was the hardest. My mom loved fruit. It gave her pleasure and satisfaction. She excluded most fruit from her diet, but since it gave her pleasure, she still ate a little. She eliminated all soda and fruit juices. Instead, she drank water with lemon. She eliminated all white flour products like bread and pasta because they are acid forming and contain refined carbohydrates that acted like sugar in her body. White potatoes and white rice were eliminated due to lack of nutritional value and the sugar spikes they cause (just like the white sugar). Potatoes and rice were staples in our home. We cooked with both most of the time. My mom couldn't believe she couldn't have white rice. We made all of our rice dishes from white rice.

All meat and dairy products had to be eliminated. The reason for this was that almost all animal products and dairy products are highly acid forming. In addition, meat and dairy products may contain steroids, antibiotics, hormones, and saturated fat. It was very hard for my mom to exclude both. She was used to eating chicken or meat almost at every meal. Both my mom and dad said that they would not be satiated if meat were not at every meal. This was going to be very hard to give up. Even then, when she could not consume a lot of food at every meal, she still loved a small piece of either chicken or a piece of steak. She said it gave her strength. Mom loved dairy products as well. She lived on yogurt, and loved eating cottage cheese with sour cream with sugar sprinkled on top.

I was not happy about telling her to stop eating the foods she loved, but because I loved her, I had to tell her to cut out her food pleasures to get better—to get rid of her cancer. You might think she would not get enough protein if she did not eat meat, but that was not true.

Beans and lentils are great alternatives to meat and are loaded with protein. Some beans are hard to digest because of their skin. Beans can cause gas, which was not an option for Mom due to the pain. There are actions you can take in order to prevent gas and help the digestion of beans. One can reduce gas and improve digestion by soaking beans overnight to and taking digestive enzymes. Many green leafy and non-leafy vegetables contain protein including zucchini, carrots, and all sprouts. I will provide a list of foods to avoid that are acidic in later in the book.

Next, we needed to figure out how to make sure Mom ingested enough greens without exhausting herself by eating them. Chewing and digestion take a lot of energy. Even a healthy person would not be able to eat as many greens as my mom needed right then. While trying to find a solution for this matter, we discovered *The Gerson® Therapy*.

Dr. Max Gerson developed the Gerson Therapy in the 1930s initially as a treatment for his own debilitating migraines, and eventually as a treatment for degenerative diseases including cancer. The

Gerson Therapy is a natural treatment that activates the body's extraordinary ability to heal itself through a plant-based diet and raw juices. The therapy utilizes a whole body approach to healing, where it naturally reactivates your body's ability to heal itself without detrimental side effects. The diet requires the daily consumption of a large amount of fresh juices containing specific nutrients, which provides the body with a super-dose of enzymes, minerals, and nutrients. All of these good substances break down the diseased body tissue, which helps our liver and kidneys to perform a natural cancer removal.

So why juice and not eat all the fruits and vegetables? There is no fiber content to the juice and, invariably, some nutrition is lost in the juicing process. An average Gerson cancer patient drinks thirteen eight-ounce glasses—about 104 ounces of fresh juice daily. This tremendous inflow of liquid provides the nutritional equivalent of almost seventeen pounds of food a day. Ingesting that quantity of food on a daily basis would be impossible. Also, most people always have difficulty properly digesting and absorbing food. This is due to toxicity, improper function of the digestive system, a decrease in stomach acid production, as well as a variety of other causes.

Dr. Gerson's clinical experimentation showed that fresh juice from raw foods both provided the easiest and most effective way to provide high quality nutrition, and produced the best clinical results.[10] He found it necessary to remove all of the bulk and fiber from the fruits and vegetables so that it was quickly and easily digested while retaining the maximum amount of nutrients and enzymes. When a person ingests juice, his or her body does not need to work hard to digest it and is maximizing the absorption of vitamins and minerals.

Why up to thirteen glasses a day? We have to understand that throughout our lives our bodies absorb a variety of carcinogens and toxic pollutants. These toxins reach us through the air we breathe, the food we eat, the medicines we take, and the water we drink. We need that amount of fresh juice (perhaps more) in order to nourish our body during a terrible sickness. Through juicing, our body undergoes an intensive detoxification regimen that eliminates these toxins from our body and it is then that the true healing process begins.

Gerson recommended that cancer patients on his therapy were to drink thirteen glasses of fresh, raw carrot or apple and green leaf juices. These juices were supposed to be prepared and drank hourly from fresh, raw fruits and vegetables. Besides juices, he also recommended three full plant-based meals freshly prepared from grown fruits, vegetables, and whole grains. The patients snacked on fresh fruit and vegetables throughout the day if they so desired.

These were drastic changes on mom's current diet. This major lifestyle shift would not be easy to implement. She was not used to eating a plant based diet, nor live solely on juices. If we wanted Mom to eat pH-balanced meals as well as apply The Gerson Therapy, I knew it would take some energy to convince her. Giving up sugar was not such a big deal. Ever since she became diabetic, she had been watching her sugar intake. The main foods that would be hard to give up would be the white stuff, like white flour, white potatoes, and so forth.

We knew it would probably be impossible for her to totally go vegan, but we tried to convince her anyway. When all components of the diet were explained to her, she cried and kept asking, "Why me?" She wanted to know why she was being punished so badly. Why did she have to get so sick? She didn't understand—she was always kind to people. She helped friends and relatives in need and always welcomed people into her warm home. It was very hard for her to understand why she couldn't eat all the comfort foods she loved. She said, "Everything that I like to eat, I can't eat with this diet. Only juice, vegetables, and fruits…and that's it? Okay. It's better to stay hungry."

We cried and laughed together about what she said. I assured her that this diet was not permanent and as soon as she got better, she could go back to the food that she loved so much. She had a comment for that. Mom always knew what to say. "Who knows if I will get better, probably not. I will die soon and die unhappy because I couldn't eat anything. So until I am alive, I will eat food that I like."

She put up a good fight for a couple of days. We changed her diet slowly adding juices. She drank four cups of juice by the end of the first week. Slowly we removed the food that was not beneficial and added more vegetarian dishes. We replaced acidic foods with alkaline foods. Slowly but surely, Mom became a vegetarian as much as was possible. It was not easy, but I was happy that she was at least trying. Mom always tried to make us feel good. She knew whatever we were doing was for her wellbeing. I am sure she appreciated it. I knew she did. Her loving eyes said it all.

Chapter 8:

Recovery — 3 Months Later

It was three months since Mom was given a short time to live, but she was still here with us, thankfully. It was amazing to see her in good spirits, have a more positive attitude toward life and actually become physically stronger little by little every day. She was still taking supplements, going for IVs twice a week, drinking juices five times a day, and eating a vegetarian diet. She stopped losing weight and actually gained a couple of pounds. The pain after she ate was not nearly as bad anymore and declined little by little every day. Her schedule was very intense and filled every minute of her day, but every day that Mom had with us was a gift.

It was the longest three months we ever had to go through. As a family, we did not know what the next day would bring—what surprise life may throw us next. Thankfully, we survived, but most importantly, Mom survived. By that time, Mom had gone through five thirty-minute treatments of body radiosurgery. The treatments were rough, but thankfully, there were only five of them and not twenty of the traditional treatments. She felt weak after each treatment, but after receiving an IV vitamin infusion, she would spring right back and feel much better.

I will never forget the day the whole family was together having a holiday meal. It was Rosh Hashana, a Jewish new year. Mom was half way through her treatment. As usual, my dad sat at the head of the table and my mom on the other end directly across from him and all their kids, son in law, and two grand kids sat all around the left and right side of them. One of the grandkids was still a baby and had her own royal chair right next to grandma.

This year, my dad helped my mom cook and I brought some dishes as well. As usual, my dad set the table to perfection. On special days like these, we used the beautiful holiday plates and glasses with silverware. We had salads, fish, and of course apples and honey to symbolize a sweet new year. Later, we served delicious main dishes and desserts. We all sat at the table so proud and happy to have our mom sitting at the table with us. We really didn't think that Mom was going to be with us for the holidays. There were beautiful toasts that brought tears and many wishes for the year to come. Everyone had exactly the same thoughts—we all wanted Mom to get well and to truly have a sweet new year!

Three months after the tall doctor relayed the stage IV metastatic cancer diagnosis, Mom saw the radiologist for another CAT scan to see if there was any change in her condition. One of the requirements after body radiosurgery is to have routine CAT scans to monitor any improvements.

Not long after, I took Mom to CINJ for a regular oncologist visit where they measured Mom's blood pressure checked her weight. Her blood pressure was normal and the scale showed weight gain. As usual, the oncologist performed a comprehensive physical exam and the was very happy to see that Mom was feeling better rather than worse. Actually, she was very surprised that Mom didn't need help getting on and off the table and was feeling stronger. We discussed Mom's diet and course of action taken for her sickness. We went over the body radiosurgery treatment Mom had and the IV infusions. The doctor did not show signs of surprise. She listened intently and did not ask questions or give her opinion.

The oncologist sat down after the physical and went over the CAT scan and blood tests completed before the visit. The blood work was good, although there were not many changes. The CAT scan results showed a reduction in the size of the tumor, although lesions in the liver and lungs were still present but did not increase in size.

When I heard the results, I went over to my mom and gave her a big hug. I could not help it, but the tears just rolled down my cheeks. This time though, they were happy tears. I looked at the oncologist and she gave us a smile. She asked if we still wanted to come for a follow up visit and if it would be ok for another doctor to take over. My mom really respected this oncologist and said to her, "You are a very good doctor. I like you. I don't want to see any other doctor." The oncologist nodded her head, said to continue with everything that Mom was doing if she felt it was helping, and then went on her way.

To tell the truth, the way this oncologist attended to my mom was very special. She was compassionate, very thorough, listened to everything we said, answered all of our questions, and was simply a lovely woman.

I know what you are going to say. Why go to the oncologist if Mom was doing treatments elsewhere especially considering that we were not using mainstream methods? Well, I thought it would be a good idea for the oncologist to continue observing my mom because I believe that the hospital and team had both the skills and tools to monitor my mom. It is not their fault they don't know certain therapies and methods. The schools, even the best ones, don't teach about alternative methods to treat cancer.

Let's face it; my mom was not their normal patient and did not succumb to the treatments she was offered. Instead, she did something that most patients don't do—and that is to take matters into her own hands with the help of her children. She took a chance and exposed her body to alternative and innovative treatments that were not very popular, which changed her fate. The body radiosurgery process was not invasive like the traditional radiation treatment, took a lot less time, and yielded superior results. During the treatment, Mom did not have to concentrate on detrimental side effects, but, instead, concentrated on her wellbeing and building her energy to fight cancer. Instead of weakening the immune system by destroying good cells together with cancer cells during traditional radiation, Mom was able to retain good cells and just kill the cancer cells with body radiosurgery, which translated to a better quality of life even during treatment.

Chapter 9:

Total Remission — 6 Months Later

Six months after the stage IV metastatic pancreatic cancer diagnosis, Mom was still alive and had outlived the three-month death sentence. Not only was she alive, but she was also in total remission. According to the CAT scan done a couple of days after the six-month mark, the big tumor at the tail of the pancreas was gone. It was a true miracle!

Mom was feeling stronger, had stamina, and was able to cook and do other chores that she had not done in a long while. She

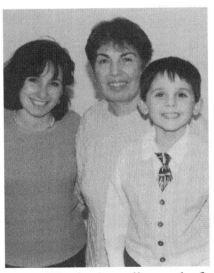 was able to take a walk outside by herself without any help. Most importantly, she was able to eat and enjoy food again. She experienced no pain after eating. She was eating because she wanted to and not because she had to for survival. Eating was not part of the schedule that she had to complete. She gained weight and looked much better. She was not pale anymore. It was strange that the littlest transitions mattered most. We don't realize and often take for granted our capability of doing it all—living life physically, intellectually, and emotionally.

Once a certain function of our body is limited, we realize how important it is.

My family is so grateful for Mom's recovery. Some of us had doubts and never thought we would have her by our side after six months. Others, including myself, always looked at the brighter side and felt grateful about the daily recovery occurring in small increments.

At this point in her recovery, mom still had a very busy schedule every day. She still ate a vegetarian diet, drank juices, took various supplements, and went for IV infusions twice a week. The protocol was still the same as before with the exception for shark cartilage. Mom begged us to get something other than the enema form (a powder and water mix) because she was tired of it. My brother discovered a liquid form of shark cartilage that became available and ordered that instead. The results were promised to be the same as the powder formula.[12] The volume of food she ate increased due to the return of her appetite. We were very happy with her progress. The diabetes she acquired still haunted her, but overall she was doing well.

Every month we went to CINJ for a visit and every time Mom passed through the doors, the nurses greeted her with a smile and were happy to see her, but were surprised that she was still alive and feeling much better. They did not have much hope. How could they when the statistics were so low? They probably saw the results of other patients that came through the same doors as my mom, which made them sad, but there was not much to do about it. When the oncologist saw Mom at the visits, she noted the improvements. Month after month, she would see Mom and would expect deterioration in her health due to the pancreatic cancer, but instead, Mom came to her office with more strength, hope, and improvement in health.

The last visit to CINJ was surprising. The oncologist greeted us the same as all the other times. During our conversation, it seemed to me that she did not want Mom to come for a subsequent monthly visit. She said that it would be sufficient to come back in six months after the next CAT scan. With confidence, the oncologist informed Mom that she looked better, gained weight, and showed overall improvement. We said goodbye and thanked her for treating my mom with respect and giving her proper care. We were truly appreciative of the knowledge she exuded during our visits and thankful that she was there for us all this time.

It's funny that the entire time that we saw the oncologist, not once did she inquire about the details of my mom's treatment—treatment that potentially could have saved many more lives and perhaps would have given other patients a second chance at life. I am actually appalled that CINJ doctors did not more actively inquire about mom's treatments and that no one wanted to know more about our process. Maybe the oncologist did her own research after she went home, but we will never know. Granted, the treatments were not FDA approved, but were effective based on prior results.

Because Mom elected to do treatments that were not FDA approved, the health insurance company did not cover 90% of the costs. Those costs became our out-of-pocket expenses. Yes, it cost a lot of money, but can you put a price on a precious life? I can't. I think life is priceless. When you want to buy a house, you take out a mortgage. In this case, you are taking out a mortgage to buy your life back. You decide how important your life is to you.

To me, the decision to spend the money was a no brainer—especially considering the 90% plus survival rate. All of the following interventions were the reason Mom was still alive after six months of being diagnosed:

- Body radiosurgery—radiation therapy that produced the least amount of side effects
- IV vitamin infusions—provided a favorable immune boost gave Mom strength and made the radiation treatments much easier to handle

- Supplements—helped strengthen the liver as well as the immune system, kill cancer cells, get rid of dead cells from the body, and help with the process of digestion

Chapter 10:

Ten Years Later

Ten wonderful years had passed since Mom was diagnosed with stage IV metastatic pancreatic cancer and had absolutely no hope of living past three months. Some people say she was lucky. Others didn't believe she had pancreatic cancer—maybe it was just pancreatitis. They say the doctors and laboratory technicians misdiagnosed the situation. After all, no one ever survived pancreatic cancer, let alone stage IV, metastatic pancreatic cancer. For a second, a doubt blew through my mind and I thought people might be right. Looking at Mom at that point made it hard to believe that she survived such a terminal illness. I kept on thinking back to the days when Mom was in such agonizing pain, couldn't eat much, and had lost so much weight that she was beyond recognition. But there was proof. A doctor performed a biopsy and a pathologist examined the tissue, which proved she had pancreatic cancer. The pathologist was in the room and looked under the microscope at the pancreas tissue to make a proper diagnosis. Other samples taken from different places in the pancreas were sent to a pathology laboratory far away for further analysis. How much more proof can there be?

I say Mom was lucky enough to make wise choices about the treatment options and other drastic dietary changes in order to combat the disease. She was lucky enough to have a strong family who cared about her and, without losing hope, did not stop at the first treatment option a doctor offered. Instead, we researched other alternative and innovative treatments that were available at the time.

Who knows, maybe we would not have the pleasure of spending all this time with Mom if we would of done it differently. Perhaps she would not have been here to see the birth of her grandson or her granddaughter. Maybe she would not have had the chance to spend quality time with her children and see her grandchildren grow and flourish through the years.

However, that is not what happened. She did get to do all those things. She thrived and lived for her husband, children, and grandchildren. She did it while having a good quality of life without any deficiencies.

Through the years, Mom traveled with her husband and sometimes family to exotic places. She went to the Caribbean Islands, Israel, Hawaii, and took local trips to the cities of the US. She always loved life and lived it to the fullest with her family at her side.

The dietary change Mom made ten years ago definitely taught her many lessons. It taught her to be more conscious about the foods she ate and how it affected her body and wellbeing. It was not really a diet for a period—it was a lifestyle change—a change that stuck with her for the rest of her life. She definitely enjoyed her food and made some modifications to her diet to include her favorite dishes of rice and meat, but she limited the amounts. Mom enjoyed birthday cakes on special occasions, but did not indulge in processed foods at all on a daily basis. She was okay with the change and did not feel deprived. After all, she is a living human being and wanted to enjoy every little bit of life every day with family, relatives, friends, and of course good food!

Mom followed the protocol of a vegetarian diet, juicing, IV infusions, and supplements for one year with a few exceptions. Nine months after the diagnosis, she added favorite dishes, but only on special occasions. Juicing was reduced to twice a day and IV infusions were reduced to twice a month. All supplements were still taken on a regular basis.

One year after the diagnosis, she maintained a 70% vegetarian diet while the other 30% was filled with mom's favorite dishes and an occasional dessert, which consisted of fruit or some baked good. She reduced juicing to once a day and IV infusions to once a month. She stopped taking shark cartilage and continued drinking Aloe Vera juice on occasion. Other supplements were still a part of her life for quite a while.

After ten years, Mom was stronger than ever. She was the head of the family, the rock again as she was before her illness, and she resumed her role. We all looked up to her for advice about anything and everything. She usually gave advice that you wanted to follow without even thinking about it. I am not sure if we just did it out of respect or because she was always right. We listened because in our minds it was the right thing to do. We always included her in all family functions. This was not because we had to, but because we wanted her to be there and to spend quality time with her. Her presence filled us with joy and happiness.

At this time, Mom's diet was unchanged from nine years before. She still adhered to a mostly vegetarian diet, which included raw and cooked vegetables, fruits, whole grains, nuts, seeds, beans, fresh herbs, and spices. She did eat white rice on occasion, which she included as part of her favorite dishes. She kept animal products such as beef, chicken, organ meats, fish, and eggs to 30% of her diet. She also reduced her intake of dairy to a minimum. As I mentioned before, Mom loved yogurt, so she ate it from time to time to satisfy her craving.

Eventually, Mom did not go for any more IV infusions and she reduced her supplements to a minimum. Even though Mom did not have cancer anymore, we still needed to make sure that she took proper supplements to prevent anything from developing in the future. She took vitamin C, fish oil, and a multivitamin daily.

Remember that your body is a very complicated machine with many functions. In order for your body to function properly and feel good, you have to take care of it and make sure to put good food into it. Otherwise, malfunction may occur and you will be at square one, the beginning, again. Our body is just like a car. We often take our car for oil changes and certain checks to make sure it runs smoothly. We also make sure to fill the car with proper fuel, otherwise the car will malfunction and not run as it once did—or not at all. Take care of it and it will take care of you. My mom understood that concept and even though she was used to eating a certain way for years, she made the changes necessary to bring her health back. We were truly blessed to have a person like my mom in our lives. To that extent, we were happy she was with us for many years against all odds.

Chapter 11:

In Retrospect

In this chapter, I would like to go back to the beginning, middle, and the end of the story to share certain experiences and answer common questions people ask me regarding my mom's sickness, treatment, and recovery.

What would you have done differently about the decision you made years ago by not going with the traditional treatment?

Based on the results, it was an easy decision. I have to say that the route that we took was the right one for my mom. People need to decide for themselves which treatment is best for their particular situation.

I can only make a deduction about traditional treatments based on the statistics of pancreatic cancer. In my mom's case, it was clear that body radiosurgery would have been the most successful treatment. Body radiosurgery yielded over a 90% survival rate, whereas traditional chemotherapy or radiation had less than 5%. There was no doubt in my mind that body radiosurgery was the only treatment for Mom. We were very happy with the results and the quality of life my mom experienced after treatment.

I would not discount the power and healing that my mom received from supplements and IV infusions. They were a very important part of the treatment that gave her strength and the necessary ammunition to face and fight the disease. I was not sure at the time if body radiosurgery would have been sufficient as a treatment by itself nor did I want to take the chance. I think we made wise decisions about everything in terms of treatment based on research at that time–I would not change anything.

Did the decisions you made impact your personal life, life with family and friends, or quality of life as a caregiver?

Before getting to the core of the question, I would like to share my experience as a caregiver, as a daughter, and as a wife and mother. Wow, those are many hats to wear. Yes, I had to juggle all of them during mom's sickness and recovery. It's very hard to see your parents suffer. It's even harder when they are young and you hear how long they have left to live. I felt like someone pushed me against a wall and did not give me any time to actually become aware of what was happening. The scenario unfolded so rapidly—everything had to happen fast. Three months was not a long time. At times, I felt numb and did not want any pain to penetrate my mind or body. The pain I felt sometimes was not the same pain my mom had although it sure seemed like it. Seeing my mom deteriorate day to day was emotionally draining.

When my mom was diagnosed with pancreatic cancer, I was living in Marlboro, New Jersey with my husband and two young children. I had a babysitter, which helped a lot, but there were still mommy responsibilities with the kids as well as household chores. Did I mention that I worked in NYC at that time as well? Yes, I worked full time. My work, my children, and my husband kept me sane through the process. When I was at work, I called my mom very often to make sure she was doing all right and following her schedule. When I came home from work after dinner and bathing my kids, I did research into the wee hours of the night. The next morning I would wake up and had to do it all over again with the exception of the days I took off from work to take my mom to the doctor or to spend time with her.

This process was physically and emotionally draining, but I had to do it. I had to be strong for my family. Thank G-d I was not alone and I had a solid support system both at home and at work. At work, I had loyal friends with whom I shared my challenges and they were willing to listen, which was helpful. I had a compassionate husband that helped at home and supported me emotionally. All of that support helped me get through this very tough time in my life.

My parents and both brothers lived in Queens. Even though they lived about an hour and a half away, our solid relationship paved the way for ease in communication, which strengthened the support system between us. We spoke often, made important decisions, and made sure that Mom always had someone with her. My brothers and father were the primary care takers for my mom. They were there at night and during the day if needed. My father and brothers worked full time and had to juggle their schedules to make sure every day was covered. We were also sensitive about making sure that each of us had some break time to do the things we needed for ourselves. Having a strong family bond really helped us stick together to make it through those hard times.

Since my mom was ill and couldn't keep the house clean by doing her regular chores, my brothers and father split the responsibilities and made sure they kept the house as clean as my mom would have. Of course that was impossible considering my mom kept everything in tip-top shape, but they tried hard. I helped when I would come over in any way I could as well.

My life turned upside down and inside out when I found out about mom's terminal illness. I had no personal life, nor was there time for friends. The only life I had was with my family. I spent my time consumed with research and determined to find a cure. Nothing else was as important. There was no time left in the day for anything else.

How did diet and all of your experiences through research influence you as a person? What changes did you adapt for yourself and your family? And why?

The information I have learned through research was invaluable. It was the key to live a healthy life. Witnessing my mom's transformation from the time of illness to recovery cannot be described in words. It was unbelievable! Watching a person recover from such a deadly disease is unthinkable, but it did happen. I believe that diet had a tremendous healing affect and helped Mom recover quicker. She only ingested nourishing and non-harming foods in her body. This made her feel good physically, mentally, and emotionally.

I became a believer in the healing process that a vegetarian diet can provide. I realized that there are many advertisements for foods that are not necessarily good for you, so I paid less attention to those and directed more attention to the labels and ingredients on the foods I ate. I became more aware that animal products, besides being highly acidic to our body, are injected with hormones and antibiotics that are then transferred to our bodies when they are ingested. Dairy products follow the same suit as they are derived from animals as well.

As I learned, I made changes within my household. The hardest part was to cut out the animal products for my family. It was much easier for me to make the change. For my husband and kids, the transformation happened gradually. At first, I started limiting the animal products we ate to five days a week, then four, and so on. Now my family has two days a week at most of animal products. I incorporated other changes as well, such as adding more fruits and vegetables to the diet—and sometimes even fresh made juices.

I believe that it is important to make lifestyle changes. They are not easy to make and sometimes feel like a sacrifice, but the change is worth it. To be and feel healthy is very important to me. For my family to be healthy is important to me as well. The importance stems from putting the right foods into our bodies and then not only feeling good, but having less visits to the doctor because of colds and other ailments that could be prevented in the first place.

How does it feel to be given a chance to heal your body and have the opportunity to live and go on living a healthy and happy life?

After recovery, this question often came up in a conversation with my mom. This is what she said, "I feel that I was given another chance to live. This is a gift. I am going to take this gift and use it well. I will continue to eat how my children have taught me. I will be healthy and spend many happy years with my family. My body has healed from an abusive disease. My mind is at peace."

Epilogue

After a full recovery, my mom lived many happy and ful-
filled years with family, relatives, and friends. Her grandchildren
really got to know her well by spending time with her and learning
about her incredible life through interviews for school research pa-
pers, different projects, and interesting trips, which made Mom very
happy.

After about 15 years, she started having stomach pains. The
pain persisted and Mom went for a checkup to a gastroenterologist
who performed an upper endoscopy. The endoscopy revealed a
stomach ulcer slightly bigger in size than on the previous test. We
knew she had an ulcer as a result of radiation treatment, but it was
under control all these years. According to results of an endoscopy
from ten years previous, the ulcer was totally healed and we thought
she had nothing to worry about.

Further tests and biopsies showed the ulcer to be malignant.
At 69 years of age, my mom was struck with stomach cancer.

My brother and I dived into research about stomach cancer
and once again found alternative treatments and supplements that
helped my mom be without pain and have a good quality of life.

Traditional treatments were offered by oncologists, but once
again, Mom did not want to go that route. I took her to surgeons that
suggested to remove the cancer, but all the research pointed to the
same amount of survival time with or without surgery. Mom decided to live whatever time she had left without any invasive treatments.

It was ironic, but three months before mom's diagnosis, I en-
rolled in the Institute for Integrative Nutrition to broaden my

knowledge about nutrition and earn a certification in Integrative Nutrition Coaching. I studied more than one hundred dietary theories and a variety of practical lifestyle teaching methods with some of the worlds top health and wellness experts. I knew there was so much I wanted to contribute to the world and other people with their health issues. I wanted to help people on a full-time basis to become healthy by eating foods that nourish the body instead of taking unnecessary medication.

With proper diet, supplementation, and alternative treatments mom lived well until about two months before she died. During those two months, her health deteriorated quickly.

Two-and-a-half years after being diagnosed with stomach cancer, mom left this world peacefully late at night.

References

[1]Somers, S. (2010). *Knockout.* New York, NY: Potter/TenSpeed/Harmony.
[2]American Cancer Society, www.cancer.org
[3]Mayo Foundation for Medical Education and Research, www.mayoclinic.org
[4]Cancer Research UK, http://www.cancerresearchuk.org/about-cancer/what-is-cancer/how-cancer-can-spread
[5]Life Extension ® http://www.lef.org//Protocols/Cancer/Cancer-Surgery/Page-04
[6]American Cancer Society, http://www.cancer.org/cancer/ pancreaticcancer/ detailedguide/pancreatic-cancer-staging
[7]Guyton, A. C., & Hall, J. (2011). *Textbook of Medical Physiology,* 783 (12th ed.). Philadelphia, PA: Saunders Elsevier.
[8]Rosenthal, J. (2014). *Integrative Nutrition.* Integrative Nutrition Publishing, Incorporated.
[9]Cook, M. S. (2008). *The Ultimate PH Solution.* New York, NY: HarperCollins Publishers.
[10]Gerson, M. (2015). Retrieved from: Gerson.org/pdfs/ Juices-for-Gerson-Therapy.pdf
[11]Warburg, O. H. (1926). *The Metabolism of Tumours,* Retrieved from: http://www.ncbi.nlm.nih.gov /pmc/articles/PMC2140820/pdf/519.pdf
[12]Lane, W. I., Comac, L. (1992). *Sharks Don't Get Cancer,* New York, NY: Avery Publishing.
[13]*The Prime Cause and Prevention of Cancer* (1931), Dr. Otto Warburg
[14]Weil, A. (2000). *Spontaneous Healing.* New York, NY: Random House Publishing Group.
[15]Weil, A. (2004). *Natural Health, Natural Healing.* New York, NY: Haughton Mifflin Harcourt.
[16]Lederman, G. (2015). Body Radiosurgery pamphlet. New York, NY. Retrieved from http://rsny.org

Your Guide to Life

In this guide I will discuss how to make necessary lifestyle changes in order for your body to heal at an optimal level thereby building a strong immune system. These lifestyle changes may need to include certain dietary changes, discipline, and strong will. I am sure you can achieve it! I will also discuss alternative treatment, supplements, and resources that pertained to my mom's recovery.

It is very important to understand the importance of eating foods that are alkaline to the body. Cancer can't survive in an alkaline environment, but thrives in an acidic environment. Here are some foods to avoid during the recovery stages and beyond if you so choose to do:

Foods to Avoid

- Dairy products – all dairy products including yogurt, goat's milk and most soy cheeses. Note: any food with the ingredient Casein is acidic.
- Meat, Poultry and Fish – it is best to eliminate during recovery due to high acidity, pesticide residue, hormones and antibiotics. Organic labels contain less toxins but still acid forming.
- White Stuff – White flour, white sugar, white rice, white potatoes.
- All processed foods such as baked goods, chips and etc.
- Canned fruits and fruit syrups.

- Alcohol including wine, beer and anything that is sweetened with juice
- All kind of soft drinks and bottled sweetened juices
- Any type of nuts and seeds that have been salted or roasted
- Corn
- Peanuts and peanut butter

Foods to Include

- All fresh vegetables
- All fresh fruits – during recovery avoid eating fruit. Later limit to 2 fruits a day.
- Whole grains – brown rice, buckwheat, quinoa, spelt
- Beans - lentils, peas, lima beans, navy beans, and soybeans
- Nuts and seeds – almonds, pumpkin and sesame seeds; make sure nuts are raw and unsalted
- Beverages – may include alkaline water and fresh vegetable juices
- Oils: olive, avocado and coconut
- Nut milk – make sure its unsweetened

Supplements

The supplements that helped mom during sickness and recovery:

- Shark Cartilage
- Milk thistle
- Reishi Mushroom Defraction
- Essaic Tea
- Enzymes

IV Infusions – please contact Dr. Michael Wald of Integrated Medicine of Mount Kisco for evaluation and suggested protocol. The contact information is as follows:

INTEGRATED MEDICINE
495 E Main Street
Mt. Kisco, NY 10549
914-242-8844
E-mail: info@intmedny.com

Body Radiosurgery – please contact Dr. Gil Lederman for more information:

RSNY – Radiosurgery New York
1384 Broadway
New York, NY 10018
212-246-4237
www.rsny.org

Meet the Author

Hi! My name is Larisa Belote and I am a Certified Integrative Nutrition Coach. During the past two and a half years, I have helped many people achieve optimal health through nutrition incorporating mind, body, and spirit into their lifestyle.

The reason I wrote this book was to give individuals with cancer hope for life. When a people hear that they have cancer, they think it's the end of the world having a deadly disease. They go to an oncologist, get scared, and jump on the first offered treatment available because that is what everyone else is doing. That is why everyone else is ending up in the same place.

Guess what? That is actually true! Or maybe that is what you hear from other people. Of course cancer is a deadly disease! Cancer does not discriminate. It can strike anyone at any age and of any race. It does not matter if you are young, old, black, or white. Just because you were told that you are going to die in a couple of months (or a year or two), don't make a quick judgment on the traditional treatments. I know you probably want to make a quick decision and start treatment right away because you are told there is no time to waste, but I want you to think about it first. Remember, it took a lot of time for cancer to grow—probably 20 to 30 years for it to form into a tumor and for symptoms to appear. I am not saying you have a lot of time on your hands, but you do have a little time to learn about your sickness and how you got it in the first place.

Please educate yourself and research other available options. When you have all the facts including all the details on traditional treatments that are available at that time, only then make an intelligent decision about the best option for your specific disease and situation. Help yourself and your body to heal at an optimal level. You will be surprised how the body can heal itself given the right tools. Learn how to rebuild your immune system so that it can fight the disease. And above all, seek support from a professional like myself who is knowledgeable in Integrative Nutrition to guide you through your step-by-step journey to recovery and optimal health.

Listen to your body. Love your mind. Get spiritual…… You are worth it!

Larisa Belote
Certified Integrative Nutrition Coach

www.stepbystep-wellness.com